Surprise!

IT'S GLUTEN-FREE!

JENNIFER FISHER

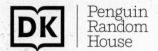

DK UK
Editor Lucy Bannell
Editorial Assistant Lucy Philpott
Senior Designer Glenda Fisher
Proofreader John Friend
Senior Production Editor Tony Phipps
Production Controller Stephanie McConnell
Jacket Designer Nicola Powling
Jacket Coordinator Lucy Philpott
Managing Editor Ruth O'Rourke
Managing Art Editor Christine Keilty
Art Director Maxine Pedliham
Publishing Director Katie Cowan

DK US
Publisher Mike Sanders
Editor Alexandra Andrzejewski
Designer and Art Director Rebecca Batchelor
Photographer Kelley Schuyler
Food Stylist Lovoni Walker
Chef Ashley Brooks
Recipe Tester Trish Sebben Malone
Proofreaders Polly Zetterberg, Lisa Himes
Indexer Brad Herriman

Picture credits
Photographs on pages 9 and 192 © Jeff Stay

All other images © Dorling Kindersley
For further information see: www.dkimages.com

First published in Great Britain in 2021 by
Dorling Kindersley Limited
DK, One Embassy Gardens, 8 Viaduct Gardens,
London, SW11 7BW

The authorised representative in the EEA is
Dorling Kindersley Verlag GmbH. Arnulfstr. 124,
80636 Munich, Germany

A CIP catalogue record for this book
is available from the British Library.
ISBN: 978-0-2414-8430-2

Printed and bound in Latvia

For the curious

www.dk.com

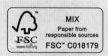

This book was made with Forest Stewardship
Council ™ certified paper – one small step in
DK's commitment to a sustainable future.

For more information go to www.dk.com/our-green-pledge

**To my boys, my biggest
fans and inspirations**

Contents

Introduction

Life revolves around food

Food is so much more than just fuel. It's intertwined with family, friendships, holidays, and memories. When I eat the same meals my parents fed me as a child – stir-fry, shepherd's pie, or chicken wings – they take my memories back decades.

When I think of gathering with family and friends for holidays, I remember the Belgian waffles with strawberries and whipped cream that my family ate every Easter morning, or the cheesy potatoes served alongside the ham at Christmas dinner. Cinnamon rolls always remind my husband of festive meals in his grandma Helen's dining room. I've even carried on my family's tradition of baking a "birthday cake for Baby Jesus" every Christmas morning.

I love how the smell and sight of certain dishes (recipes for many of which are in this book) flood me with nostalgia. There are more than 100 recipes in *Surprise! It's Gluten-Free!*, and almost all of them have deeply rooted ties to my family and friends, the incredible people who originally started making these recipes over the years. I've turned their tried-and-tested dishes into gluten-free renditions. If you or someone for whom you cook has a gluten allergy, or wants to change their eating habits, then these gluten-free recipes are for you. I hope you find joy, tradition, and comfort in the same foods that are so important to me.

Cooking: it's in my DNA

I developed a love for cooking at a very young age. My mum was always whipping up great treats in the kitchen, whether it was for a birthday, a holiday, or just a family Sunday lunch, and I loved spending time in the kitchen with her.

I can remember making peanut butter balls and rolling them in a dozen different coatings, or helping my mum to recreate family staples to be cholesterol-friendly for my father, that tasted just like the amazing original recipes. Cooking was a bonding activity that always produced delicious results.

Not only do I love to cook anything and everything, but I have also always had a deep love for all baking: cream puffs (mum made the best), pies (again, mum's apple pie can't be beaten), cakes (it's why I go to weddings), and doughnuts (oh my, *doughnuts!*). I was a child who always wanted waffles for breakfast, or cinnamon rolls, or anything else that involved bread or dough. For lunch and dinner, I always went for pizza, pasta, rice… all foods that were big on carbs. I would eat at certain restaurants because of the bread they served before the meal. Little did I know, all these foods had a grave effect on my body.

Mysterious symptoms

For the first 22 years of my life, I had never heard the word "gluten". In my early twenties, I began to experience debilitating symptoms that affected my day-to-day life. I had no explanation for them and not the slightest idea they were tied to gluten, but they lasted for years. Severe anxiety, panic attacks, crippling gastrointestinal (GI) upset, daily headaches or migraines, constant mouth ulcers, joint pain, persistent nausea, cramping, body aches, extreme fatigue, weight loss, and brain fog… these were my normal. I was afraid to go to sleep at night for fear of waking up an hour later, sick to my stomach. I was even scared to leave my house after dinner, developing something called agoraphobia, an anxiety disorder characterized by extreme fear of public places.

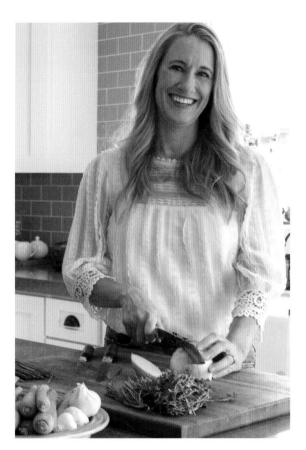
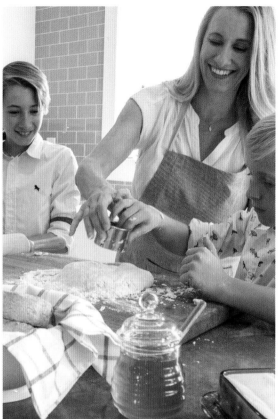
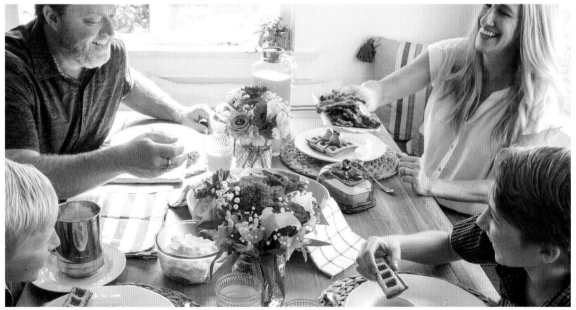

I sought medical help and underwent *so* many tests, none of which revealed any clear insight into what was wrong. When I started to stumble upon the unfamiliar words "gluten" and "coeliac" associated with a list of symptoms that matched my own, my doctors were dismissive. At the time, coeliac disease and gluten sensitivity were poorly understood in the mainstream medical community, and as a result, I was lumped into the general diagnosis of irritable bowel syndrome (IBS) and told to try yoga and find other ways to relieve stress.

Any time I thought I'd found the solution to my years of pain and uncertainty, more medication would be thrown my way and my symptoms would improve slightly… then I would have a bad flare-up, receive a round of steroids, and start all over again.

As a young adult, I was barely able to manage my symptoms. I continued looking for answers, and every time I researched, I would come across gluten and coeliac disease. Although my symptoms matched, my doctors would say, "No, that's not it." They also advised, "Don't give up gluten. In fact, eat more whole wheat. It's good for your colon."

I had decided that this was my life: weird diets, constant research, and the prospect that I would live out the rest of my days feeling sick and defined by my anxiety.

Change for good
I remained resigned to what I had come to believe was my fate until I had kids. That changed everything, and I recommitted to fighting for my health. I wanted to be "active mum", "fun mum", and "spontaneous mum". I had a friend and mentor who was a nutritionist and natural wellness practitioner in my town, so I set up an appointment with her, and the first thing she told me was to stop eating gluten (a term that was ever-so-slowly becoming a household word).

Oh my goodness! My life changed. My health changed. Within months, my headaches were gone, my heavy-feeling body was light, my foggy brain was clear, and all my joint pain subsided. I'm still healing from years of damage, but my severe GI symptoms have gone away. My life definitely changed when I cut out gluten, and I have never looked back.

Good food, but make it gluten-free
Going gluten-free was extremely hard for me because traditional, gluten-containing foods had been central to my diet. However, the alternative (eating gluten and feeling awful) was so much worse than the lifestyle change. I know because I've "cheated" a few times and paid the price in misery.

I officially went gluten-free in 2008, when there were very few gluten-free alternatives on the supermarket shelves, and most restaurants had no idea how to cater for a growing generation of gluten-free diners. On the rare occasion I did find gluten-free snacks or bakes in a shop, they were outrageously expensive, and I would often throw them out anyway, because they fell so disappointingly short of the tastes and textures I loved in their gluten-filled counterparts.

After spending unsustainable amounts of money on food I wasn't eating, I decided to use my love of cooking in a new way. My mother had bestowed on me a strong culinary instinct, and I knew it was time to start experimenting and creating all the foods I was missing.

I can't tell you how many flour combinations I tried or how many loaves of bread or batches of cookies went straight into the bin; if it tasted or looked gluten-free, then it was back to the drawing board. Eventually though, I got the hang of it. There are so many techniques and ingredients I've discovered throughout the process, and I'm really proud of the gluten-free dishes that have come out of my kitchen. If my personal taste testers – my family – are any testimony, then you could call my gluten-free creations a raving success.

The persistent experimentation turned into a small side business for me. I started baking for a few local stores and farmers' markets in San Clemente, California, and began my own company, JF Bakes. My creations had a growing positive reputation. I started meeting strangers who found out I was the baker of "the best pumpkin bread" they'd ever had. Shop owners wanted more of my goods on their shelves. I learned just how well-loved my baking was.

Turning the page

My business grew fast, as did my two young boys, and I became overwhelmingly busy. I decided I couldn't juggle both professional baking and being the mum I wanted to be, so I closed the company. Shortly after, my older son Max was diagnosed with gluten sensitivity. This inspired me to keep cooking and creating, because I wanted him to have all the same meals and treats that every other child around him was enjoying.

One of the traditions at our family Thanksgiving meal is Grandma Helen's Cinnamon Rolls. There was no way I was going to let those rolls be passed around under Max's nose without him enjoying one. So, I took up the task of creating a gluten-free cinnamon roll that he and I could both enjoy, and now you can too, by following the recipe on page 36. The first few times we went to theme parks after he became gluten-free, we would walk past the churros stands and inhale the heavenly smell of fried dough with cinnamon and sugar. So, the next day we would make gluten-free churros and eat until our hearts and tummies were content. I never want my children to miss out on these food memories that last a lifetime.

When people ask me what my passions are, what makes me smile and get excited, it's easy to answer: seeing a child eat a cupcake, or a cookie, or a muffin for the very first time. I love it when I create a treat my son hasn't been able to eat in years and his face absolutely lights up when he takes his first bite. Or when someone is shocked that what they're eating is gluten-free: that's my passion.

That is also why I'm writing this book. My hope is that the recipes in these pages will enable you and your family and friends to enjoy delicious foods with full confidence that they support your health.

I want you to escape the hassle of cooking two of everything, one with gluten and one without. Now you can serve all your family and friends the same tasty home-cooked meals and desserts without one of them ever guessing that what they're eating is gluten-free. Please, just remember to say: "Surprise! It's gluten-free!"

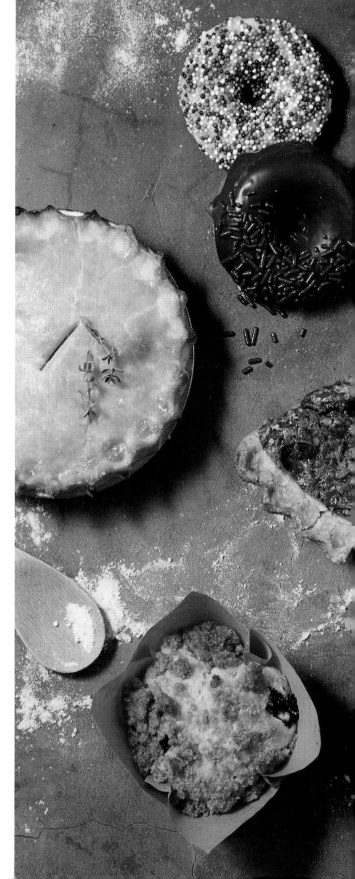

Gluten-Free Basics & Essential Flour Blends

Gluten Explained

Baking is a science that must be performed precisely. If, for health reasons, you need to remove gluten from your baking, the science becomes even trickier, approaching more of an art form. There are no hard-and-fast rules for how to remove gluten-containing wheat from your breads and cakes and still get the structured, airy products you've always loved. However, we can look at all the ways that gluten makes your food amazing, compensate with alternative ingredients, and throw in a whole lot of trial and error in the test lab (my kitchen). You should be able to take a bite and never know what was missing.

From hero to villain

Gluten is a protein that gives baked goods structure, elasticity, and a light texture. When you use it in batters and doughs, it creates little air pockets and then acts like a miraculous net throughout a dough to trap bubbles, resulting in the airy, beautiful crumb you see when you slice into a loaf. This effect can be difficult to replicate in gluten-free baking. Gluten seems to be the magic ingredient for amazing baking… plus maybe you've heard that grains are part of a healthy, balanced diet.

However, those with coeliac disease, gluten sensitivity, and other autoimmune conditions have a hard time processing gluten. When someone with these illnesses eats a food containing gluten, their immune system goes into overdrive and begins to attack their own tissues. This causes inflammation throughout the body, which leads to joint pain, skin reactions, gastrointestinal upset, nutritional deficiencies, and more. These are debilitating symptoms, and for those with coeliac disease specifically, gluten causes long-term damage to the small intestine, making it a very disruptive villain to the body's systems.

The only way to eliminate the symptoms is to completely remove gluten from your diet. This is a significant lifestyle shift, but a worthwhile pursuit when you find your symptoms are managed, or even disappear. If gluten is disrupting your life like it did mine, it's time to plunge into the world of gluten-free alternatives. You probably already know that shop-bought gluten-free foods can be expensive and less than delicious, so I'm thrilled to begin truly fantastic gluten-free baking with you.

The art of gluten-free baking

When you remove gluten from baking, the main challenge is creating a product that isn't dense, dry, or gritty, or that sinks in the middle, or crumbles to pieces upon the first bite. To make matters more difficult, techniques and ingredients that work for one gluten-free recipe might not work for the next. To imitate gluten, we add emulsifiers and stabilizers to baking, along with alternative proteins and starches. Ingredients such as rice flour, tapioca starch, eggs, and vinegar work together to create beautiful, bubbly baking that you'd never know was gluten-free! I've done all the hard work for you with meticulously tested recipes that withstand the criticism of the most sceptical taste buds.

Once you start baking with gluten-free flours and living a gluten-free lifestyle, the easier it becomes. One of the easiest ways to always be prepared for gluten-free baking is to keep a large batch of my all-purpose gluten-free flour blends (see p24) on hand. These will become your go-to flours. With my many other secret tricks and ingredients, you'll soon master this art form.

Gluten-containing grains

When you're avoiding gluten, you need to know all the foods that contain it. It's not just wheat flour that you need to watch out for. Gluten is the protein found in all wheat, rye, and barley. There are over 30,000 wheat varieties grown throughout the world. Some of the more common varieties are spelt, farro, durum, kamut, bulgur, farina, semolina, and einkorn. Oats are also always in question.

While they are naturally free of gluten, oats are often grown or packed close to wheat, so cross-contamination can occur, which makes them irritating for many people. When you buy oats, confirm they're certified gluten-free.

The same principle applies to all other packaged goods: make sure you see an explicit certification of gluten-free; otherwise, you risk cross-contamination, which can be okay if your symptoms are more subtle, but will wreak havoc on individuals who are extremely sensitive. Some products may have the label "wheat-free", but you need to confirm that they don't contain other forms of gluten from rye, barley, malt, or oats. You will soon learn that gluten is everywhere – in salad dressings, sauces, spice mixes, marinades, even cosmetics – but with practice, you'll learn how to read labels, ask questions, and discern whether a product is safe for you.

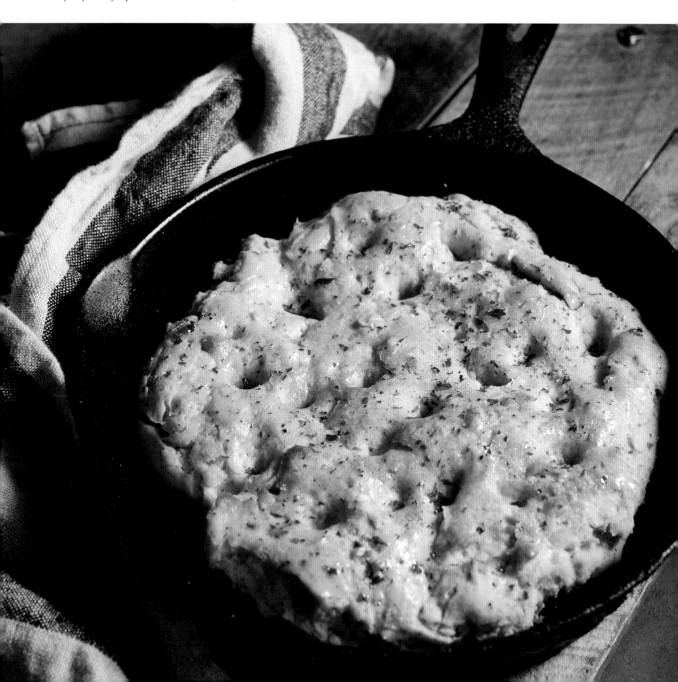

Secret Ingredients

Before you head into the kitchen to start baking your first batch of gluten-free goodies, take a little time to read about the ingredients and tips that make these recipes extra-special. The specific ingredients I discuss here help to create fluffier bakes that hold together well and will not crumble to pieces. I use these in almost every single one of my recipes to create textures that leave everyone questioning whether or not my baking is really gluten-free.

Flours

The million-dollar question: what do you use for flour when you can't use wheat flour? The answer is: a blend of many different ingredients. You can't use just one flour alternative (such as only rice flour, or solely ground almonds) as a one-for-one substitute for wheat flour; you'll need to combine a few different grains and starches to reach the desired effect. I have created three different flour blends that use some combination of these ingredients: white and brown rice flour, tapioca flour, potato starch, arrowroot, sorghum flour, teff flour, and ground almonds. I usually try to buy flours that are both organic and certified gluten-free, as I find them to be of the highest quality.

- **Arrowroot** (also called *arrowroot powder)* is an easily digested starch from the arrowroot plant. Unlike most other starches, it's actually high in protein and several other nutrients.

- **Brown rice flour** is denser than other gluten-free flours, which is why it's best used in blends. It's ground from the whole grain, preserving the bran and germ from the rice kernel. It has a mild, nutty flavour and is high in fibre, protein, and B vitamins.

- **Ground almonds** are made from blanched almonds (not the same as almond meal, which is coarser and contains the ground skins). They have a light, sweet flavour and keep baked goods moist; they are low-carb, nutrient-rich, and high in fat and protein.

- **Potato starch** adds moistness to gluten-free baking. It's the starch extracted from potatoes and is not the same thing as potato flour (which is flour ground from whole potatoes). This is also a great thickening agent for soups and sauces.

- **Sorghum flour** has a light colour and texture with a mild, sweet flavour. It's a good source of protein, iron, B vitamins, fibre, and antioxidants.

- **Tapioca flour** (also called *tapioca starch)* is a pure starch from the cassava root. It's excellent for thickening soups and sauces and has a slightly sweet flavour.

- **Teff flour** works best when blended with other flours and starches, as it has a very distinct flavour. It's high in calcium, protein, and iron, and it contains an excellent balance of amino acids.

- **White rice flour** imparts slight sweetness and a smooth texture.

Binders

I use xanthan gum in nearly all of my baking. It's a food additive produced by a microorganism called *Xanthomonas campestris*. Xanthan gum helps create elasticity in dough and batter, acting as a gluten substitute to bind all the ingredients together. Although xanthan gum is not absolutely necessary, without it, your bakes will have a more crumbly texture and tend to fall apart after baking. I don't add xanthan gum to my pre-mixed flour blends, as I use differing amounts in each recipe.

Note that large amounts of xanthan gum (anything over about 15g/½oz daily) may have a laxative effect or cause digestive discomfort. Most of my recipes use only 3–9g (less than ¼oz), and you're likely to eat only a few servings of any recipe in one day. However, if you have digestive issues with xanthan gum, consider using an identical amount of guar gum (another thickening agent), instead. I have used both and have no preference for one over the other. My suggestion is to use whichever your body tolerates best.

Eggs

Many of my recipes rely on eggs (always large ones). They are important for binding in gluten-free baking and help your recipes hold their structure. I use organic eggs in my baking and cooking. You could try using egg substitutes if you're sensitive to eggs, but these will not yield the same outcome and may cause your bakes to crumble.

Leavening agents

Baking powder increases the volume and lightens up your bakes; perfect for when you're working with gluten-free flours. I always use aluminium-free versions. A few of my recipes call for bicarbonate of soda as well, but because bicarbonate of soda requires acid to activate, it's only included in recipes with a higher acid content. Always check the expiration dates on the packages.

Sugars

You'll notice I always call for golden granulated sugar, which is unrefined. Unlike refined sugar, it isn't pure white in colour and the crystals are a bit larger. You can substitute with refined white sugar, but it may not always yield the same result.

You can substitute coconut sugar in any recipe, gram-for-gram. Maple sugar may be substituted as well, however it's twice as sweet as golden granulated sugar, so you may need to experiment to get to a sweetness level you prefer. I don't recommend using honey or maple syrup in place of sugar, as the wet-to-dry ingredient ratio will be out of balance and may not produce a good result.

Apple cider vinegar

If you've ever picked up a loaf of gluten-free bread or a gluten-free cake, you might have noticed it's quite heavy. Gluten-free baked goods tend to be very dense, but apple cider vinegar helps lighten them up. When mixed with bicarbonate of soda, it creates tiny bubbles of carbon dioxide gas in your dough, which produces fluffier, lighter mixtures that rise a little better and won't sink. I always use apple cider vinegar that contains the "mother", the active enzyme component of vinegar that makes it look a little cloudy but imparts many health benefits. I recommend you also always choose a raw, unfiltered vinegar that contains the "mother", or your results may differ.

Butter

Any salted butter will work, but I prefer to use organic butter made from the milk of grass-fed cows. Please consider using a high-quality butter such as this, if it's available, because it makes a notable difference to the flavour of your baking.

Maintaining a gluten-free lifestyle

Beginning a gluten-free diet can be daunting and may seem impossible, but I promise it gets easier with time. I don't give it a second thought any more because it's so much a part of how I live. Here are my top tips for success:

- **READ LABELS!** Gluten is sneaky.

- **FULLY STOCK YOUR GLUTEN-FREE KITCHEN.** Always have a gluten-free flour blend prepared and stored in the refrigerator. Other helpful staples are gluten-free condiments, pasta, and chicken stock. Tamari (gluten-free soy sauce) or coconut aminos are great soy sauce substitutes to have.

- **NEVER ASSUME A MENU ITEM IS GLUTEN-FREE.** Always alert the waiter to your allergy. Many people are so sensitive they can't eat anything that has been fried in the same oil that was used for a product containing gluten. For example, I can only eat chips or crisps if they have been fried in their own oil, not oil used for chicken nuggets, battered fish, or any other item containing gluten.

- **CARRY SNACKS EVERYWHERE YOU GO.** I usually have gluten-free crackers, a piece of fruit, or a gluten-free mini salami in my handbag.

- **CHECK YOUR TOILETRIES.** Not everyone is sensitive to this, but if you are, double-check every product. (It's surprising how much shampoo actually rinses into your mouth!) If you're eating gluten-free and not seeing relief in your symptoms, this is the next place to check.

- **BE WARY OF CROSS-CONTAMINATION.** If you're sharing a kitchen where gluten is used, be careful of work surfaces and utensils. For example, don't stir a pot of regular spaghetti and then use the same spoon to stir your gluten-free pasta. Also, flour travels through the air very easily. If wheat flour was previously used in your kitchen, be sure to clean any work surfaces, utensils, or appliances before making anything gluten-free.

- **CHECK YOUR MEDICATION.** Gluten is often used as a binder in medicines or tablets.

- **TRY TO COOK AT HOME AS MUCH AS POSSIBLE.** Not only is it safer, because you know exactly what is in your food, but it will help your wallet, too. Gluten-free foods can be very expensive, especially when eating out. You will almost always notice a price increase when choosing a gluten-free burger bun or pizza dough.

- **DON'T CHEAT!** A gluten-free diet is unlike any other; you can't have a "cheat day" every so often, or you will not find relief from your symptoms. Gluten stays in your body for a long time. For example, if I accidentally eat gluten, it often takes weeks before I feel normal again. If you notice you're not getting any better on a gluten-free diet, make sure you're not accidentally consuming gluten somewhere; even the smallest amounts can affect sensitive people.

- **IF YOUR FAMILY IS SUPPORTIVE, MAKE YOUR WHOLE HOUSE GLUTEN-FREE.** We've done this in my house even though only two out of the four of us must avoid gluten. First, this makes life easier. It can be very taxing to cook multiple meals every day. Second, it helps you avoid cross-contamination. I don't want wheat flour touching my appliances. Third, it's cheaper. Buying many versions of breads, pastas, or crackers can be very expensive. Finally, it improves your gluten-free cooking skills!

Using shop-bought flour blends

I'll be giving you the recipes for the flour blends I use in every recipe in this book (see p24). If you don't have the time or desire to mix up these blends, you can use a ready-made shop-bought blend. But, when choosing products, look for something that is similar to one of my recipes. I cannot guarantee you'll arrive at the same final result, but they should work. However, substituting straight rice flour or oat flour (or any single type of gluten-free flour) will not work. In order to create the elasticity, structure, and proper texture, you need a certain amount of starch combined with the flours. Blends always work the best!

Other fats & oils

I often use hard white vegetable fat in my baking, which creates a tender crumb and a crispy crust. However, not all fats are created equal. The amount of water can vary between brands, which can cause your baked goods to come out differently. For instance, if you use a brand with a higher water content, your dozen cookies could spread into one mega-cookie! I always use organic white vegetable fat and recommend that you use it as well. If you are not able to find it, try using butter instead, or refrigerate both your white vegetable fat and your dough before baking, to stop your bakes spreading excessively.

For cooking and baking with oil, avocado oil is my favourite. It has a very light flavour and the highest smoke point of all plant-based oils; unlike others, it won't oxidate when heated to high temperatures, which is thought to be toxic for your body.

Pasta

Try to find the Doves Farm brand, if possible. If I can't find this brand, then I will use any variety of 100 per cent brown rice pasta, which I've found is the most similar to wheat pasta; it holds its shape and has the best texture. In my experience, pastas that include corn or other grains tend to crumble, or can be crunchy, especially if not eaten immediately.

I have two tips for cooking with gluten-free pasta. First, never cook it for as long as the package says; I usually start tasting it 3–4 minutes before the recommended cooking time is up. Second, rinse the pasta under water immediately after cooking. This will wash off the starches and help prevent the pasta from becoming slimy or mushy. The recipe will specify if you need to use hot or cold water.

Milk

I use organic whole milk or canned full-fat coconut milk in most of my recipes that call for milk. You can substitute almond milk, rice milk, or canned full-fat coconut milk in place of cow's milk in any recipe. Some recipes call for canned coconut cream, by which I mean the solid, thicker part of the full-fat canned coconut milk, but you can substitute double cream.

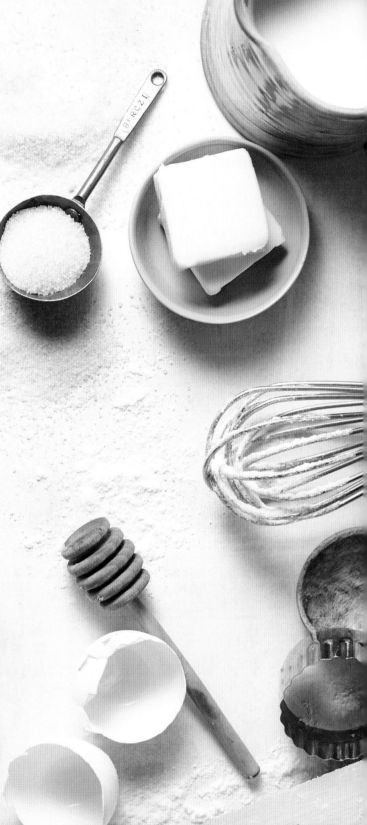

Secret Techniques

Gluten-free baking is often about trial and error. Fortunately, I've done all the trial and error for you. If you follow recipe methods precisely, measure ingredients properly, and use the suggested brands, you too can have baked goods that taste just like the gluten-filled originals!

Measuring

Careful measuring, especially of flour and flour blends, is very important in baking, and I recommend that you always use accurate scales. Digital scales are the most exact, but you can use manual, too. For both types, make sure the scales are set to zero before weighing the ingredients. If you are using measuring spoons for the smaller quantities (teaspoons and tablespoons), the best way is to overfill them and then level off with a knife (see photo). You don't need to sift flour or flour blends for my recipes, unless specifically instructed.

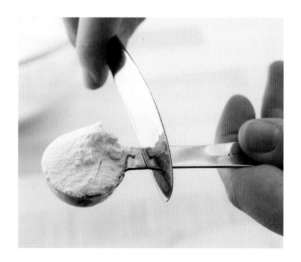

Greasing

You'll notice most of my recipes instruct you to only grease the base of the tin (not the sides). Gluten-free bakes need all the help they can get to achieve a proper rise, and the sides of the tin give doughs and batters something to stick to, helping your bakes keep their risen shape. If the sides are greased, the dough tends to pull away from them and then sink. Once your bakes are cooled, if they need a little bit of coaxing out of the tin, you can gently run a butter knife around the inside.

Mixing time

Because there is no gluten in your dough, in general you don't need to be cautious of overmixing (which in conventional baking risks overdeveloping the gluten) or undermixing. But there are still some occasions when mixing time is important. For instance, if you overmix scones, they will not be flaky. If you overmix a recipe containing whipped egg whites, the batter could deflate. For recipes with yeast, you need a few minutes of extra mixing (to take the place of kneading). For the best success, always follow the recipe instructions.

Kneading doughs

Gluten-free doughs are very different from doughs with gluten, especially bread doughs. They will be much stickier and thinner, and you won't be able to knead a gluten-free dough as you would a dough containing gluten. My recipes all call for "kneading" your dough using a stand mixer fitted with the paddle attachment. The doughs are too thin and sticky for the hook attachment.

Flouring work surfaces

Because the doughs are so much stickier, any time you place the dough on a work surface, it's very important that you've floured it properly. I almost always choose baking parchment as a base, and usually use tapioca flour when flouring surfaces; it tends to work the best in preventing sticking to the work surface and it also blends in nicely with the dough without leaving a gritty layer on the final product, as rice flour would. You could also use a flour blend, but there would be a slight risk of drying the mixture out too much.

Freshness of ingredients

Fresh ingredients are critical and may be the reason for a disappointing bake. For example, baking powder is used to create rise and lighten the texture of your baking; expired baking powder could cause a cake or muffin to sink. The same is true of bicarbonate of soda, yeast, and eggs.

Temperature of ingredients

Some recipes call for firm (chilled), softened, or room temperature butter, eggs, or white vegetable fat. It's critical to follow the directions when they specifically mention at what temperature the ingredients should be, or your baking may not turn out as it should, often due to excessive spreading. When a recipe uses yeast, it is likewise very important to add warm water within the specified temperature range, or the yeast might not activate.

Baking in batches

When baking cookies, muffins, scones, or anything else on a baking tray, only cook one tray at a time, in the middle of the oven, with the items properly spaced apart on that tray. Your baked goods won't cook evenly if the oven is overcrowded. For most of my recipes, you'll need to bake in batches. However, gluten-free batters tend to get fluffier the longer they sit, so cooking in batches is usually a good thing. (The muffins or cupcakes from the last batch always have the best crown on them, because they get to sit the longest before going in the oven!) Keep an eye out, though, for certain recipes that require refrigeration between batches.

Allowing batters & doughs to rest

Resting allows flours and starches to absorb moisture, which will soften the mixture and create more of a rise in your baking. You'll get the best structure and shape if you follow instructions for resting (and sometimes chilling or freezing) doughs.

Cooling

Because gluten-free goods tend to be a bit more delicate than their counterparts, you'll often see instructions to cool your food on or in the tin instead of removing it to a rack. Do not rush or skip this part! Removing your baking from its tin too quickly may result in a pile of crumbs at worst, or a sunken disappointment at best.

Read the recipe all the way through before starting

Some recipes call for ingredients at room temperature, or for chilling before baking. You don't want to start a cookie recipe that you plan to eat right after dinner and then realize the dough needs to chill for hours!

Storing foods

Fresh gluten-free bakes tend to dry out much faster than a gluten- or preservative-filled item, and refrigeration often accelerates the drying out process. I very rarely suggest storing any of your baking in the refrigerator. Gluten-free items are best stored in the freezer. The freezer helps retain their moisture and prevents them from drying out. However, it is very important that your items are placed in an airtight container or freezer bag first. I like to separate each serving with baking parchment or cling film, as well.

Troubleshooting

Here are some common errors and how to address them.

- **NO "CROWN" ON MUFFINS, CAKES, OR CUPCAKES:** There are many factors to consider. Check the freshness of baking powder and bicarbonate of soda. If you have too much liquid in a mixture, increase the flour 1 tablespoon at a time. An oven that is too hot can cause the item to set before the bubbles have formed a rise; if the oven is too cold, the item will rise too quickly and then fall before the centre has set. You need a slow and consistent rise, so always preheat the oven thoroughly, and consider double-checking its temperature with an oven thermometer. If butter or white vegetable fat is too soft, refrigerate the batter before baking to help the food rise in the oven, instead of melting.

- **DRY OR CRUMBLY:** If a mixture has too much flour, add liquid 1 tablespoon at a time. If you didn't use xanthan gum when it was called for, that may also cause crumbliness. Finally, overcooking will give a drier final product.

- **GUMMY OR DENSE:** If gummy, you may have used too much xanthan gum. (But hopefully my recipe testing has prevented denseness!) If you're still having trouble, check the freshness on your baking powder or bicarbonate of soda, or use a bit more. Omitting any apple cider vinegar will also lead to a denser product.

- **ALTITUDE ADJUSTMENTS:** Baking at higher altitudes can be difficult, particularly when you throw "gluten-free" into the mix. I've found that the following tips help create a great final product. **(1)** Increase oven temperature by 10°C (15°F), and reduce the baking time by 5–8 minutes. **(2)** Increase the flour by 1 tablespoon for every 125g (4½oz). **(3)** Reduce sugar by 1 tablespoon for every 200g (7oz). **(4)** Increase the liquid by 1–2 tablespoons (or add 1 additional egg white). **(5)** Reduce the baking powder and bicarbonate of soda. (This part is tricky; go carefully and look for advice online, too.)

- **MUSHY IN THE MIDDLE:** Your food was either not cooked long enough or had too much liquid in the batter.

- **SPREADING EXCESSIVELY:** You either have too much liquid in the dough, or your dough needs to be refrigerated before baking.

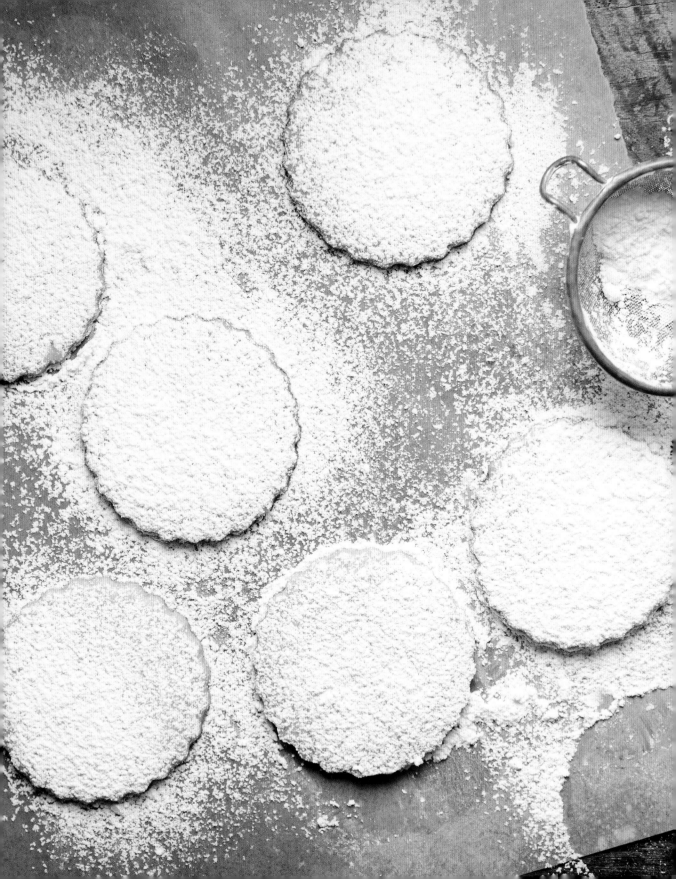

The Blends

Whip up a batch or two of my amazing flour blends and keep in the refrigerator, making gluten-free baking a cinch. My favourite is the No. 1 All-Purpose Flour Blend, which tends to be very forgiving, but the No. 2 All-Purpose Flour Blend is great for sensitive tummies. The Ancient Grain Flour Blend is ideal when you have a fancy for something that tastes whole grain.

No. 1 All-Purpose Flour Blend

This is the flour blend I use most often. I make a large batch of it and store it in an airtight container in my refrigerator. It can easily replace white flour in almost any recipe gram-for-gram. I also use this if a recipe calls for flour to thicken a sauce. It is a great all-purpose flour.

Yield
about 675g (1½lb)

300g (10oz) white rice flour
200g (7oz) brown rice flour
100g (3½oz) tapioca flour
75g (2½oz) potato starch

No. 2 All-Purpose Flour Blend

This is another all-purpose blend that I use in a few of my recipes. It's made without brown rice flour. I almost always use my No. 1 All-Purpose Flour Blend, but if you do not digest brown rice very well, then use this version as a substitute in any recipe.

Yield
about 700g (1½lb)

500g (1lb 2oz) white rice flour
110g (3¾oz) potato starch
35g (1¼oz) arrowroot
70g (2¼oz) tapioca flour

Ancient Grain Flour Blend

Unlike modern wheat, corn, and white rice, ancient grains are a grouping of crops that haven't been changed (or only very slightly altered) by selective breeding. This blend is a great wholemeal flour replacement. It has a higher protein, fibre, antioxidant, and vitamin content than my other two flour blends. It's also moister than the other blends and may require longer cooking times. The final product is typically a bit denser.

Yield
about 1kg (2lb 4oz)

200g (7oz) sorghum flour
300g (10oz) brown rice flour
200g (7oz) teff flour
125g (4½oz) arrowroot
175g (6oz) tapioca flour

For any of the blends, in a large bowl, whisk or sift all the flours thoroughly to combine, making sure the blend is evenly mixed.

Store it
Keep in an airtight container at room temperature for 1–2 months, in the refrigerator for 4–6 months, or in the freezer for up to 1 year.

Tip
I recommend using digital kitchen scales to measure out the different flours. While not essential, it's the best way to create an accurate blend. If you don't have digital scales, be sure to measure the flour as exactly as possible, or it will not create a good blend.

Home-Made Breadcrumbs

I have used many different brands of shop-bought plain gluten-free breadcrumbs over the years. Some have been fantastic and others no good at all. The problems I have run into are always related to texture: they are either dry and hard, or they can be the exact opposite and turn mushy as soon as they come into contact with any moisture. When in a hurry, shop-bought gluten-free breadcrumbs will work in any of my recipes, but if you have the time, home-made breadcrumbs create better texture and flavour. They are very easy to make and store very well in an airtight container in the freezer. So, before you throw out any stale gluten-free bread, use it to make breadcrumbs and then toss them in the freezer, ready to pull out and use at any time.

Yield
about 75g (2½oz)

4 slices of gluten-free bread

1. Preheat the oven to 180°C (160°C fan/350°F/Gas 4). Cut the bread slices into 2.5cm (1in) cubes. Arrange the cubes in a single layer on a baking tray.

2. Bake for 15 minutes. If the bread is still soft at all, continue to bake for 5–10 minutes, checking often to make sure it doesn't burn.

3. Cool the bread cubes and then pulse in a food processor until fine crumbs are formed.

Store it
Store in an airtight container in the freezer for up to 6 months.

Tip
Use your favourite shop-bought gluten-free bread, or use home-made bread. Good options from this book include Traditional English Muffins (see p31), Ancient Grain Sandwich Bread (see p112), Easy White Sandwich Bread (see p113), and Hamburger Buns (see p116). I like to collect all the odds and ends of bread that no one eats and keep them all in a bag in the freezer. Once I've collected a good amount, I use them to make breadcrumbs.

Wheat-Free Mornings

Makes:
18-24

Prep time:
10 minutes, plus cooling

Cook time:
30 minutes

70g (2¼oz) flaked or slivered almonds

35g (1¼oz) sunflower seeds

30g (1oz) pumpkin seeds

200g (7oz) rolled oats (certified gluten-free)

25g (1oz) desiccated coconut

80g (2¾oz) No. 1 All-Purpose Flour Blend or Ancient Grain Flour Blend (see p24)

½ tsp xanthan gum

½ tsp ground cinnamon

40g (1¼oz) salted butter

75g (2½oz) raw honey

115g (4oz) pure maple syrup

45g (1½oz) coconut sugar

1½ tsp vanilla extract

¼ tsp salt

85g (3oz) finely chopped pitted dates

85g (3oz) finely chopped dried apricots

75g (2½oz) dried cranberries or raisins

My Oat Bars (see p176) – which are a surefire crowd-pleaser and definitely a dessert – inspired this lightly sweetened breakfast recipe. A few friends asked me for a healthier version of those oat bars, so I created these, which do not contain any refined sugar and are full of delicious, healthy ingredients.

Chewy Granola Bars

1. Preheat the oven to 180°C (160°C fan/350°F/Gas 4) and line a 30 x 20cm (12 x 8in) or 33 x 23cm (13 x 9in) baking tray with baking parchment.

2. Put the almonds, sunflower seeds, and pumpkin seeds in a food processor and pulse a few times, just enough to chop them up a little bit.

3. In a large bowl, stir together the chopped nuts and seeds, oats, and coconut. Spread the mixture out on to a separate baking tray. Bake for 10–12 minutes, stirring occasionally, until lightly toasted.

4. Transfer to a large bowl and mix in the No. 1 All-Purpose Flour Blend, or Ancient Grain Flour Blend, xanthan gum, and cinnamon. Reduce the oven temperature to 150°C (130°C fan/300°F/Gas 2).

5. In a small saucepan, stir together the butter, honey, maple syrup, coconut sugar, vanilla, and salt, and bring to the boil over a medium heat. Once it starts to boil, cook, stirring constantly, for 1 minute.

6. Pour the hot mixture over the oat mixture. Add the dates, apricots, and cranberries, and stir well. With wet fingers, to prevent the mixture from sticking to your hands, spread the mixture into the parchment-lined baking tray and press down until evenly spread.

7. Bake for 20–25 minutes or until starting to turn light golden brown. Cool in the pan for at least 2–3 hours before cutting into 7.5cm (3in) long bars.

Tips

Refrigerate the dates and apricots for a few hours before making these bars, to make them easier to chop.

If you have a hard time digesting nuts or seeds, you can soak them in filtered water for about 4 hours before starting this recipe. Soaked nuts and seeds are more easily digested.

Mix it up with your choice of dried fruits or nuts. For example, replace the dates, apricots, or cranberries with dried apples, cherries, blueberries, or pineapple.

For extra luxuriousness, drizzle melted chocolate on top of the cooled bars.

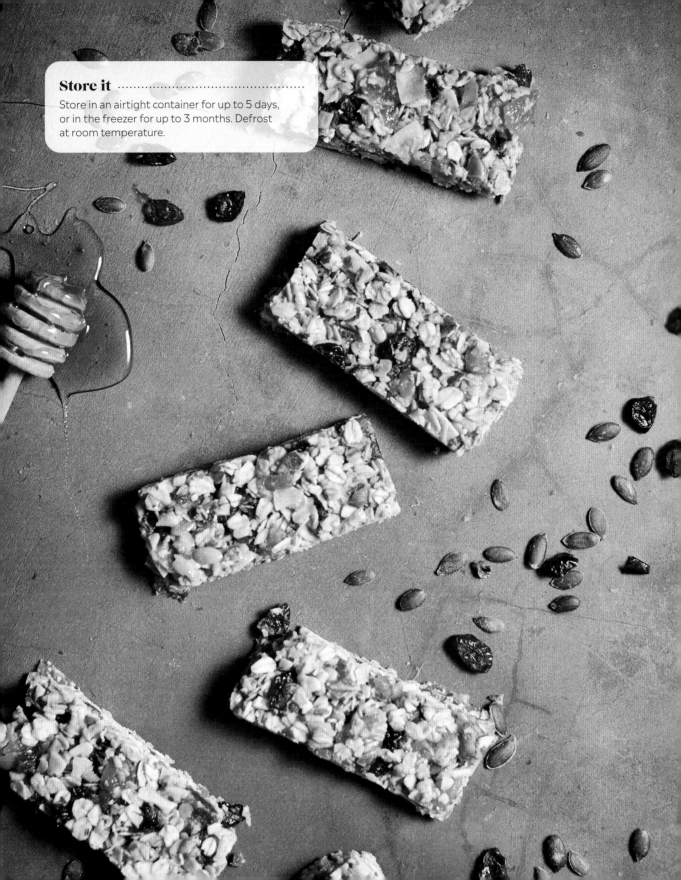

Store it ·····································

Store in an airtight container for up to 5 days,
or in the freezer for up to 3 months. Defrost
at room temperature.

Makes:
about 675g (1½lb)

Prep time:
10 minutes, plus cooling

Cook time:
55 minutes

I developed this lightly sweet, crunchy, nut-filled granola when I was looking for a healthier option containing more than just oats. When I was baking and selling to a few local shops, it quickly became a customer favourite. It's great with ice cream, or mixed with the topping on an apple or berry crumble.

Almond Granola

90g (3¼oz) flaked or slivered almonds

100g (3½oz) sunflower seeds

100g (3½oz) pumpkin seeds

175g (6oz) rolled oats (certified gluten-free)

75g (2½oz) desiccated coconut

1 tsp ground cinnamon

½ tsp salt

80g (2¾oz) coconut oil, melted

35g (1¼oz) raw honey

60ml (2fl oz) filtered water

1 tsp vanilla extract

1. Preheat the oven to 150°C (130°C fan/300°F/Gas 2) and line a large baking tray with baking parchment. In a large bowl, combine the almonds, sunflower seeds, pumpkin seeds, oats, coconut, cinnamon, and salt.

2. Add the melted coconut oil to the items in the bowl and stir to evenly coat. Warm the honey in the microwave for about 20 seconds to melt it slightly, and then add to the mixture and stir again until well combined.

3. In a small bowl, stir together the water and vanilla. Add to the granola and stir well. Evenly spread the granola on the prepared baking tray, spreading it to the edges and levelling it as much as possible.

4. Bake for 45–55 minutes, stirring the granola every 10 minutes for the first 30 minutes, and then every 5 minutes for the remaining cooking time. Be sure to smooth the granola back out after each stir. It is ready when it turns golden brown. Cool completely on the baking tray and serve at room temperature.

Store it ....
Store in an airtight container for up to 2 weeks, or in the freezer for up to 3 months. Defrost at room temperature.

Makes:
6

Prep time:
1 hour, plus 45 minutes to rise, and cooling

Cook time:
35 minutes

Special equipment:
cooking thermometer

320ml (11fl oz) whole milk

1 tbsp golden granulated sugar

1 tsp salt

15g (½oz) salted butter

2 tsp apple cider vinegar

120g (4½oz) white rice flour

65g (2¼oz) tapioca flour

135g (4¾oz) Ancient Grain Flour Blend (see p24)

2 tsp xanthan gum

2¼ tsp fast-action dried yeast

a little flavourless oil

cooking spray, for coating

50g (1¾oz) ground almonds, for sprinkling

Store it ....

These muffins freeze very well without drying out. Split them apart before freezing, then put them back together and individually wrap in cling film. Freeze in an airtight container. When ready to eat, you can either place directly into the toaster, defrost at room temperature, or in the microwave for 20–30 seconds.

Any kind of toasted bread with butter is my favourite morning snack, and these English muffins fit the bill. Don't let the number of cooking steps overwhelm you; they're really easy to make, so prepare a double batch and keep some in the freezer. You'll need six English muffin rings.

Traditional English Muffins

1. In a small saucepan, combine the milk, sugar, salt, and butter over a low heat. Stir until the sugar is dissolved. Transfer the mixture to a stand mixer fitted with the paddle attachment, or a large bowl. Let cool to 41–43°C (105–110°F). Once the milk reaches the specified temperature range, stir in the vinegar.

2. While the milk mixture is cooling, sift together the rice flour, tapioca flour, Ancient Grain Flour Blend, xanthan gum, and yeast. Add the flour blend to the milk, and beat on low speed until well incorporated. Scrape down the sides of the bowl. Beat again on medium-high speed for 3 minutes. The dough will be very sticky. Cover and set aside in a warm place to rise for 30–45 minutes or until doubled in size. When it has risen, gently stir the dough with a spatula to deflate.

3. While the dough is rising, preheat the oven to 180°C (160°C fan/350°F/Gas 4). During the last 5 minutes of rising, heat a frying pan over a medium-low heat. Lightly oil the pan. Spray the insides of six English muffin rings with cooking spray and set together on the warm pan.

4. Sprinkle about 1 teaspoon of ground almonds onto the pan inside each ring. Scoop about 85g (3oz) of dough into each ring. Spray the top of each muffin with cooking spray. Place a piece of baking parchment over the rings and lightly press the dough down with a spoon to smooth. Remove the parchment. Sprinkle about 1 teaspoon of ground almonds on top of each muffin, then return the baking parchment to the top. Place a baking tray on top of the baking parchment-covered rings to prevent them from rising too much.

5. Cook for 4–6 minutes or until lightly golden brown on the bottom. Uncover and use two spatulas to flip the rings. Re-cover with the parchment and baking tray, and cook for another 4–6 minutes. Transfer the rings to another baking parchment-lined baking tray and bake in the oven for 3 minutes. Remove the rings from the muffins, place a new piece of baking parchment on top of the muffins, along with a baking tray if needed to prevent the paper from curling. Bake for 15 minutes more, or until the edges spring back when pinched.

6. Cool on a wire rack for 10–15 minutes. When cool enough to touch, use a fork to perforate the muffins all around the perimeter. The dough will be very gooey on the inside, and you will need to clean your fork during the process. When ready to eat, cut the muffins in half and toast. They can be used for eggs Benedict, or topped with butter, jam, almond butter, or your favourite topping.

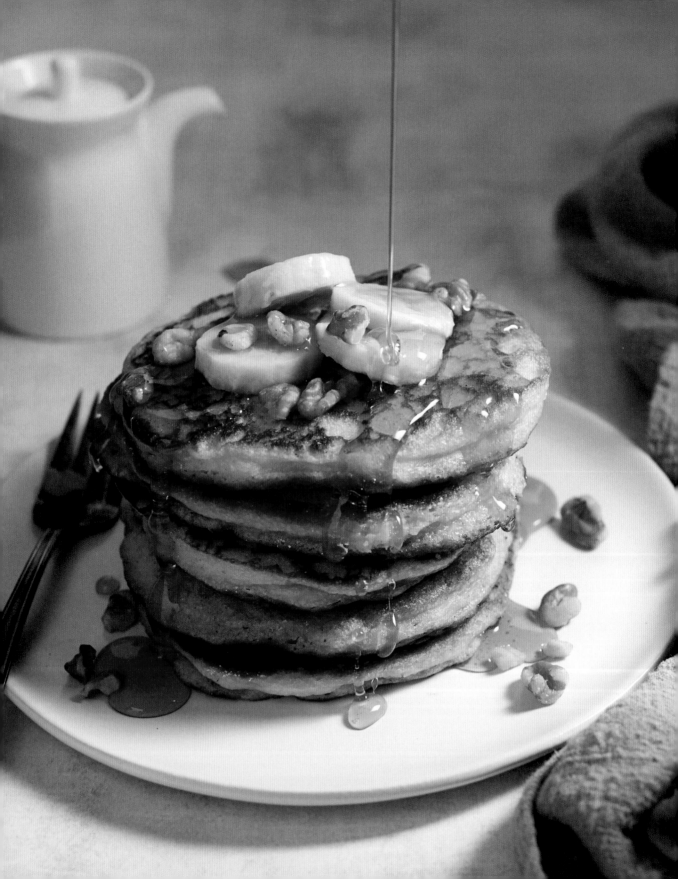

Makes:
12 x 7.5cm (3in) diameter pancakes

Prep time:
10 minutes

Cook time:
10 minutes

240ml (8fl oz) whole milk, plus extra if needed

1 tbsp lemon juice

160g (5¾oz) No. 1 All-Purpose Flour Blend (see p24)

1 tsp xanthan gum

2 tbsp golden granulated sugar

1 tsp baking powder

½ tsp bicarbonate of soda

½ tsp salt

1 large egg

1 tsp vanilla extract

30g (1oz) salted butter, melted and cooled

white vegetable fat or coconut oil, for greasing

butter, pure maple syrup, banana slices, walnuts, chocolate chips, berries, or icing sugar, to serve (optional)

My children would eat pancakes every single morning if I put a stack in front of them, so creating a super-delicious wheat-free pancake recipe was a must. I love serving these to people who aren't gluten-conscious, because they have no idea they are gluten-free!

Fluffy Pancakes

1. In a small bowl, whisk together the milk and lemon juice and set aside for 5 minutes to sour.

2. In a large bowl, whisk together the No. 1 All-Purpose Flour Blend, xanthan gum, sugar, baking powder, bicarbonate of soda, and salt.

3. In a separate medium bowl, lightly beat the egg. Whisk in the vanilla, soured milk, and melted butter. Pour the milk mixture into the flour mixture and whisk until smooth.

4. Heat a non-stick frying pan over a medium heat, and then grease it with vegetable fat or coconut oil. Ladle scoops of batter onto the preheated pan and cook for 1–2 minutes or until golden brown on the bottom. (You will have to cook these in batches.) Flip and cook until golden brown on the other side. Note that pancake batter may thicken as it sits. If it gets too thick to work with, add small amounts of milk, 1 tablespoon at a time, to thin it out.

5. Serve immediately with butter, pure maple syrup, banana slices, and walnuts, or any other topping of your choice.

Store it

Cool on a wire rack. Place in an airtight container with sheets of baking parchment separating the pancakes. Freeze for up to 3 months. When ready to eat, place directly into the toaster.

Tips

The lemon juice is the secret to the fluffiness of these pancakes. It reacts with the bicarbonate of soda, creating tiny air bubbles that fluff up the batter.

To make these a bit healthier, prepare a version using the Ancient Grain Flour Blend. For the flour, use 100g (3½oz) Ancient Grain Flour Blend and 40g (1¼oz) No. 1 All-Purpose Flour Blend (see p24). You could also replace the golden granulated sugar with coconut sugar.

These are great breakfast waffles to eat before heading out to school or work. They are full of nutrient-dense grains and oats. Keep a large batch in the freezer and pop them into the toaster in the morning to reheat. Greasing the waffle iron with white vegetable fat is a must to create the crispy outer crust.

Ancient Grain Waffles

melted white vegetable fat, for greasing

200g (7oz) Ancient Grain Flour Blend (see p24)

25g (scant 1oz) ground almonds

1 tsp xanthan gum

3 tbsp coconut sugar or maple sugar

25g (scant 1oz) rolled oats (certified gluten-free)

2 tsp baking powder

1 tsp salt

½ tsp bicarbonate of soda

360ml (12fl oz) whole milk

2 tsp apple cider vinegar

1 tsp vanilla extract

45g (1½oz) salted butter, melted and cooled, plus extra (optional) to serve

2 large eggs, separated

maple syrup or fresh fruit, to serve (optional)

1. Preheat the waffle iron according to the manufacturer's instructions and lightly brush it with vegetable fat.

2. In a large bowl, whisk together the Ancient Grain Flour Blend, ground almonds, xanthan gum, coconut sugar, oats, baking powder, salt, and bicarbonate of soda until thoroughly combined.

3. In a medium bowl, whisk together the milk, vinegar, vanilla, and butter. Put the egg whites into a separate medium bowl. Add the yolks to the milk mixture and then whisk until well combined. Whisk these wet ingredients into the dry ingredients until just homogenous, but do not overmix.

4. Beat the egg whites until soft peaks form. Gently fold the egg whites into the batter.

5. Ladle some of the batter into the prepared waffle iron and cook according to the manufacturer's instructions. These waffles tend to spread out, so do not fill too full or manually spread out the batter too much. Brush more vegetable fat onto the waffle iron between batches. Serve warm with butter, maple syrup, or fruit.

Store it

Let the waffles cool completely on a wire rack. Place in an airtight container with baking parchment separating the waffles. Freeze for up to 3 months. When ready to eat, place directly into the toaster.

Makes:
5–6

Prep time:
20 minutes

Cook time:
15 minutes

melted white vegetable fat, for greasing

2 tbsp lemon juice

480ml (16fl oz) whole milk

320g (11oz) No. 1 All-Purpose Flour Blend (see p24)

1 tsp xanthan gum

2 tbsp golden granulated sugar

2 tsp baking powder

1 tsp bicarbonate of soda

½ tsp salt

3 large eggs, separated

75g (2½oz) salted butter, melted and cooled, plus extra (optional) to serve

1 tsp vanilla extract

maple syrup or strawberries and whipped cream to serve (optional)

For the whipped cream (optional)

250ml (9fl oz) double cream

1–3 tbsp pure maple syrup, to taste

Growing up, we would have Belgian waffles with strawberries and whipped cream every Easter morning, so a good home-made waffle recipe was absolutely vital! Your morning guests will all love these little luxuries and won't miss a thing.

Belgian Waffle Wannabes

1. Preheat the waffle iron according to the manufacturer's instructions and lightly brush with vegetable fat. In a medium bowl, whisk together the lemon juice and milk, and set aside for 5 minutes to sour.

2. In a large bowl, whisk together the No. 1 All-Purpose Flour Blend, xanthan gum, sugar, baking powder, bicarbonate of soda, and salt until well combined.

3. Put the egg whites into a separate medium bowl. Add the yolks to the soured milk, along with the melted butter and vanilla and whisk until well combined and frothy. Add the milk mixture to the flour mixture, and whisk until just homogenous.

4. Beat the egg whites until soft peaks form. Gently fold the egg whites into the batter.

5. If you're making the whipped cream, in a stand mixer fitted with the whisk attachment, or in a medium bowl, beat the cream with the maple syrup until stiff peaks form.

6. Ladle some of the batter into the prepared waffle iron and cook according to the manufacturer's instructions. Brush more vegetable fat onto the waffle iron between batches. Serve warm with butter, maple syrup, or strawberries and whipped cream (if desired).

Store it

Let the waffles cool completely on a wire rack. Place in an airtight container with baking parchment separating the waffles. Freeze for up to 3 months. When ready to eat, place directly into the toaster.

Makes:
8–9

Prep time:
30 minutes, plus
2 hours to rise, and
cooling

Cook time:
25 minutes

Special equipment:
cooking thermometer

60g (2oz) salted butter,
softened, plus extra
for greasing
240g (8½oz) No. 1
All-Purpose Flour Blend
(see p24)
160g (5¾oz) sorghum
flour
65–100g (2¼–3½oz)
tapioca flour, plus extra
for dusting
2¼ tsp fast-action dried
yeast
2 tsp xanthan gum
1 tsp salt
1 tsp powdered gelatine
100g (3½oz) golden
granulated sugar
2 large eggs
240ml (8fl oz) warm water
at 41–43°C (105–110°F)
1 tbsp apple cider vinegar

For the filling

60g (2oz) salted butter,
melted, plus extra
(optional) to serve
85g (3oz) light brown
sugar
2 tsp ground cinnamon

For the icing (optional)

130g (4½oz) icing sugar
½ tsp vanilla extract
2–2½ tbsp whole milk

These cinnamon rolls are a firm tradition in my husband's family. We made a trip to see 92-year-old Grandma Helen and she showed me how it's done. I adapted her recipe to be gluten-free and now we all get to enjoy her rolls.

Grandma Helen's Cinnamon Rolls

1. Lightly grease only the base of a 20 or 23cm (8 or 9in) square baking tin. In a medium bowl, stir together the No. 1 All-Purpose Flour Blend, sorghum flour, 65g (2¼oz) of the tapioca flour, the yeast, xanthan gum, salt, and gelatine.

2. In a stand mixer fitted with the paddle attachment, or in a large bowl, cream together the butter and sugar on medium-high speed until light and fluffy. Add the eggs one at a time, blending well on high speed after each addition, then add the warm water and vinegar and blend on medium speed until combined.

3. Slowly add the flour mixture to the wet ingredients and beat on low speed until combined. Increase the speed to medium-high and beat for 2 minutes. The dough will be very sticky. If it's too sticky to get out of the bowl, add tapioca flour 1 tablespoon at a time, but do not add more than 100g (3½oz) in total.

4. Heavily dust a 60cm (2ft) long sheet of baking parchment with tapioca flour. Wet your hands with warm water and spread the dough over the length and width of the parchment, making it 45–48cm (18–19in) long and 3–5mm (⅛–¼in) thick. Continue to wet your hands while pressing out the dough to prevent sticking.

5. For the filling, brush the melted butter over the dough from edge to edge. In a small bowl, combine the brown sugar and cinnamon. Sprinkle over the dough from edge to edge.

6. Starting at a short side, and using the parchment as a guide, very carefully roll up the dough as tightly as possible, patching any holes by squeezing the dough together. Using a sharp knife dipped in tapioca flour, cut the roll into 9 equally sized discs, and place into the prepared baking tin cut sides up. (It's fine if they touch.) Let them rise in a warm place for 1–2 hours or until almost doubled in size. When they're almost ready, preheat the oven to 190°C (170°C fan/375°F/ Gas 5).

7. Bake for 20–25 minutes or until starting to turn golden brown. Cool in the tin until the butter stops bubbling, and then flip them out onto a plate. Serve warm with butter, or ice them.

8. If using icing, stir the icing sugar in a bowl with the vanilla and 2 tablespoons of milk. Add more milk 1 teaspoon at a time as needed until a smooth, thin icing is formed. Drizzle this over the cooled buns and leave to set.

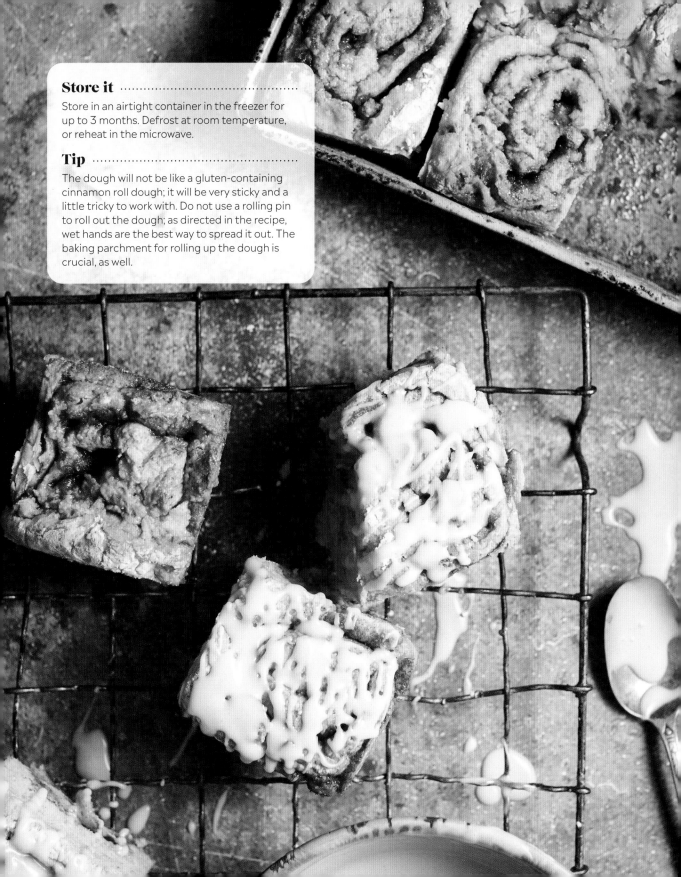

Store it ....

Store in an airtight container in the freezer for up to 3 months. Defrost at room temperature, or reheat in the microwave.

Tip ....

The dough will not be like a gluten-containing cinnamon roll dough; it will be very sticky and a little tricky to work with. Do not use a rolling pin to roll out the dough; as directed in the recipe, wet hands are the best way to spread it out. The baking parchment for rolling up the dough is crucial, as well.

Makes:
about 10

Prep time:
15 minutes, plus cooling

Cook time:
15 minutes

320g (11oz) No. 1
    All-Purpose Flour Blend
    (see p24), plus extra for
    dusting, if needed

2 tsp xanthan gum

2 tsp baking powder

1 tsp bicarbonate of soda

1 tbsp golden granulated
    sugar

½ tsp salt

70g (2¼oz) white
    vegetable fat

1 tsp apple cider vinegar

240ml (8fl oz) sour cream

1 large egg

1 tbsp water

butter, honey, or jam,
    to serve

These are amazing eaten warm in the morning. Or my mum makes exceptional Oven "Fried" Chicken (see p58 for my version) and often serves it when we come over for Sunday lunch. These light and flaky savoury scones go hand-in-hand with fried chicken, too!

Flaky Sour Cream Scones

1. Preheat the oven to 220°C (200°C fan/425°F/Gas 7) and line a baking tray with baking parchment. In a medium bowl, whisk together the No. 1 All-Purpose Flour Blend, xanthan gum, baking powder, bicarbonate of soda, sugar, and salt until combined.

2. Using a pastry cutter or fork, cut the fat into the dry ingredients until pea-sized crumbs are formed.

3. In a small bowl, stir together the vinegar and sour cream. Using a wooden spoon, stir the mixture into the dry ingredients until just barely combined.

4. Turn the dough onto a work surface lined with baking parchment. The dough will be very crumbly, so squeeze it together until it holds the shape of a ball. It will have cracks in it. (If the dough becomes sticky, flour your hands.) In order to create flaky scones, do not overwork the dough.

5. Gently press the dough into a disc about 2.5cm (1in) thick. Cut out the scones using a biscuit cutter about 6.5cm (2½in) in diameter. Continue gathering and shaping the scraps and cutting out scones until you have used all the dough.

6. In a small bowl, lightly beat together the egg and water. Brush the top of the scones with the egg wash.

7. Place the scones on the prepared baking tray and bake for 15 minutes, or until lightly brown on top. Let cool on the baking tray for a few minutes. Serve warm with butter, honey, or jam.

Store it

Store in an airtight container for up to 2 days, or in the freezer for up to 3 months. Defrost at room temperature.

Tip

If you use a brand of white vegetable fat with a high water content, you may find your scones excessively spreading. If you're unsure about your brand of fat, chill the dough for at least 1 hour before baking, to help prevent them spreading.

Makes:
6–8

Prep time:
45 minutes, plus
45 minutes to rise

Cook time:
15 minutes

Special equipment:
cooking thermometer

560g (1¼lb) No. 2
   All-Purpose Flour Blend
   (see p24), plus extra
   for dusting
2 tsp xanthan gum
¼ tsp salt
1 tbsp fast-action dried
   yeast
300ml (10fl oz) whole milk
2 large eggs, at room
   temperature
1 tbsp apple cider vinegar
35g (1¼oz) golden
   granulated sugar, plus
   extra for coating
115g (4oz) salted butter,
   melted
140g (5oz) Pastry
   Cream Filling (see
   p165, steps 1–2)
high smoke-point oil
   (such as avocado oil),
   for deep-frying

Store it

Store in an airtight
container in the freezer
for up to 3 months.
Defrost at room
temperature.

Tips

These are great with
Chocolate Glaze (see
p40) drizzled on top.

You can also make them
jam-filled by replacing
the Pastry Cream Filling
with your favourite jam.

These are the closest thing to a doughnut-shop doughnut I have ever had. The creamy centre helps create an incredibly light and moist doughnut. You do not need a deep-fryer – a frying pan works – although I do recommend the investment; it's worth it just for these!

Cream-Filled Doughnuts

1. In a medium bowl, stir together the No. 2 All-Purpose Flour Blend, xanthan gum, salt, and yeast. Set aside.

2. Over a low heat or in the microwave, warm the milk to 41–43°C (105–110°F).

3. In a stand mixer fitted with the paddle attachment, or in a large bowl, lightly beat the eggs on medium speed. Add the warmed milk, vinegar, sugar, and butter, and beat on medium-low speed until combined.

4. Add the flour mixture to the milk mixture, and beat slowly on low speed to combine. Slowly increase the speed to medium and beat for 3 minutes more.

5. Turn the dough onto a well-floured surface. The dough will be very sticky and not as pliable as gluten-containing dough, so make sure you use plenty of flour.

6. Flour the top of the dough. Roll the dough out until 1cm (½in) thick. Use a 6–7.5cm (2½–3in) round biscuit cutter to cut out doughnuts. Continue gathering and shaping the scraps and cutting doughnuts until you use all the dough.

7. Transfer the doughnuts to a baking parchment-lined baking tray and cover with another sheet of baking parchment. Set in a warm place to rise for 30–45 minutes or until doubled in size.

8. While the doughnuts are rising, make the Pastry Cream Filling (see p165, steps 1–2). Set aside in the refrigerator until ready to use.

9. In a deep-fryer or in a heavy-based deep saucepan with oil about 7.5cm (3in) deep, preheat the oil to 180°C (360°F). If the oil is too cold, the doughnuts will absorb too much and become heavy and greasy. If it's too hot, the doughnuts will brown too quickly and not be cooked through in the middle. Fill a shallow dish with golden granulated sugar for rolling the doughnuts in after frying.

10. Once the doughnuts have doubled in size and the oil is hot, carefully place 1 or 2 at a time into the hot oil. Fry for 1–1½ minutes, and then flip. Fry for 1 minute more, and then remove. Let the doughnuts cool on a wire rack for just a minute or so, until cool enough to touch but still slightly hot. While the doughnuts are still warm, roll them in the sugar and then set on a wire rack to cool for 10–15 minutes. Repeat until all the doughnuts are fried and coated.

11. Once the doughnuts have cooled, poke a hole on one side of each that goes to about the middle. (A chopstick works really well for this, or a thin sharp knife.) Fill a squeeze bottle or piping bag with the Pastry Cream Filling. Squeeze it into each doughnut until plump. These are best served the same day.

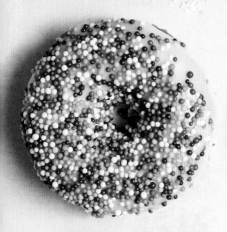

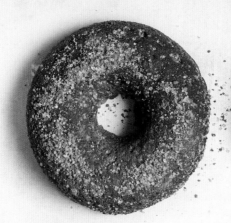

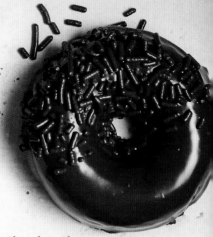

Vanilla Glaze:

60g (2oz) salted butter, melted
1 tsp vanilla extract
1 tsp golden syrup
400g (14oz) icing sugar
80–120ml (2½–4fl oz) whole milk
sprinkles (optional), for decorating

In a medium bowl, stir the butter, vanilla, syrup, and icing sugar until smooth. Add 80ml (2½fl oz) milk and stir until smooth. Add more milk 1 tablespoon at a time until a thin icing forms. Dip the top of the cooled doughnuts in the glaze, and top with sprinkles (if using). Set on a wire rack until the glaze hardens.

Cinnamon Sugar:

100g (3½oz) golden granulated sugar
85g (3oz) light brown sugar
1 tbsp ground cinnamon
45g (1½oz) salted butter, melted

In a bowl, combine both sugars and the cinnamon. Brush the cooled doughnuts lightly with melted butter, then roll in the cinnamon-sugar mix until well coated.

Chocolate Glaze:

200g (7oz) icing sugar
4 tbsp cocoa powder
3 tbsp whole milk
1 tsp vanilla extract
1 tsp golden syrup
sprinkles (optional), for decorating

In a medium bowl, whisk together the icing sugar and cocoa powder. Slowly stir in the milk, vanilla, and syrup, and whisk until smooth. Dip the top half of the cooled doughnuts in the glaze and top with sprinkles (if using). Set on a wire rack until the glaze hardens.

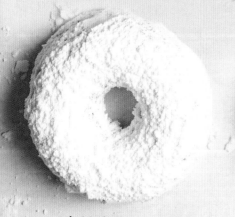

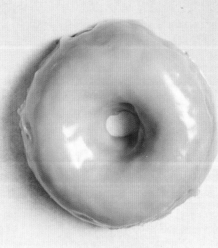

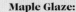

Maple Glaze:

60g (2oz) salted butter
1 tsp golden syrup
115g (4oz) pure maple syrup
130g (4¾oz) icing sugar

In a small saucepan over a low heat, stir together the butter, golden syrup, and maple syrup. Once melted, remove from the heat and whisk in the icing sugar. Let cool and thicken slightly. Dip the top half of the cooled doughnuts in the glaze. Set on a wire rack until the glaze hardens.

Icing Sugar:

260g (9oz) icing sugar

Place the icing sugar in a shallow dish. As soon as the doughnuts are cool enough to touch (but still very warm), roll them around in icing sugar until well coated. Once cooled, re-roll them once or twice more.

Makes:
30 mini doughnuts
or 10 full-sized

Prep time:
20 minutes, plus cooling
and decorating

Cook time:
15 minutes

160g (5¾oz) No. 1
    All-Purpose Flour Blend
    (see p24)
1 tsp xanthan gum
150g (5½oz) golden
    granulated sugar
½ tsp bicarbonate of soda
1 tsp baking powder
¼ tsp salt
1 large egg
120ml (4fl oz) whole milk
1 tsp apple cider vinegar
1 tsp vanilla extract
30g (1oz) salted butter,
    melted, plus extra
    (optional), for greasing
cooking spray (optional),
    for greasing

If I was asked, "What's the first thing you'd eat if you could have gluten again?" hands down my response would be "a DOUGHNUT!" I'm not sure I'll ever eat a shop-bought doughnut again, but these satisfy my cravings. Choose one variety, or make all five! This is best in a doughnut maker, but if baking them, I recommend silicone moulds.

Doughnuts 5 Ways

1. If using the oven instead of a doughnut maker, preheat the oven to 180°C (160°C fan/350°F/Gas 4). In a large bowl, whisk together the No. 1 All-Purpose Flour Blend, xanthan gum, sugar, bicarbonate of soda, baking powder, and salt.

2. In a separate medium bowl, lightly beat the egg. Add the milk, vinegar, vanilla, and melted butter, and beat until well combined.

3. Pour the wet ingredients into the dry ingredients and whisk until a thick, smooth batter forms. Let the batter sit for 5–10 minutes.

4. If using a doughnut maker, preheat it and grease. If using a doughnut tin in the oven, spray the moulds with non-stick cooking spray.

5. Pour the batter into a piping bag or a resealable plastic bag. Cut the tip off the icing bag or one corner off the plastic bag. Pipe the batter into the greased doughnut maker or doughnut tin, filling each mould two-thirds full.

6. Bake in the doughnut maker for 3–5 minutes (or according to the manufacturer's instructions), or bake in the oven for 12–15 minutes or until golden brown.

7. Let cool on a wire rack (and in the doughnut tin, if used) while preparing your desired toppings. If you are making icing sugar doughnuts, roll them as soon as they're cool enough to touch.

Store it

Once completely cooled, store in an airtight container for 2-3 days or freeze for 2-3 months. Separate layers of doughnuts with baking parchment. Defrost in a single layer at room temperature.

Tips

The longer the batter sits, the fluffier the doughnuts will be. Prepare the batter up to 1 hour ahead of time.

Each topping recipe is enough for 1 batch (30 mini doughnuts or 10 full-sized doughnuts). Plan your quantities accordingly if you'd like a variety of doughnuts.

These doughnuts can be adapted for every occasion by changing the sprinkles you put on top: orange and black for Halloween; or pink, red, and white for Valentine's day.

Fish & Poultry Mains

The light flavour and flakiness of halibut makes it my favourite fish, and this macadamia nut crust adds such a delicious twist. The mango salsa pairs just perfectly with this recipe. I always try to buy fresh halibut, but when it's not available, I go for frozen skinned halibut fillets, which work just as well.

Macadamia Nut Crusted Halibut
with Mango Salsa

80g (2¾oz) No. 1 All-Purpose Flour Blend (see p24)

2 large eggs

100g (3½oz) chopped, roasted, and salted macadamia nuts (processed until finely chopped)

1 tbsp chopped flat-leaf parsley

¼ tsp garlic powder

½ tsp salt

⅛ tsp freshly ground black pepper

2 tbsp desiccated coconut

25g (scant 1oz) Home-Made Breadcrumbs (see p25) or shop-bought plain gluten-free breadcrumbs

4 halibut fillets, about 225g (8oz) each

For the salsa

165g (6oz) chopped mango

3 tbsp chopped red onion

3 tbsp chopped coriander

2 spring onions, chopped

¼–½ jalapeño, to taste, finely chopped

juice of 1 lime

salt and freshly ground black pepper

1. Preheat the oven to 200°C (180°C fan/400°F/Gas 6) and line a baking tray with baking parchment. Put the No. 1 All-Purpose Flour Blend in a shallow bowl or on a large plate. In a second shallow bowl, lightly beat the eggs. In a third shallow bowl or another large plate, stir together the macadamia nuts, parsley, garlic powder, salt, pepper, coconut, and breadcrumbs.

2. Dredge the fish fillets in the flour blend, shaking off excess. Then dip into the eggs. Finally coat in the nut mixture, pressing the fish firmly down to coat all sides thoroughly. Carefully place the fillets onto the prepared baking tray.

3. Bake for 20–25 minutes or until the fillets are golden brown, no longer opaque in the centre, and flake easily. If the macadamia crust starts to get too brown before the fish is fully cooked, cover with a piece of baking parchment.

4. Meanwhile, make the salsa. In a small bowl, stir together the mango, red onion, coriander, spring onions, jalapeño, lime juice, salt, and pepper. Refrigerate until ready to use.

5. Serve the halibut as soon as it is cooked, with the mango salsa on top.

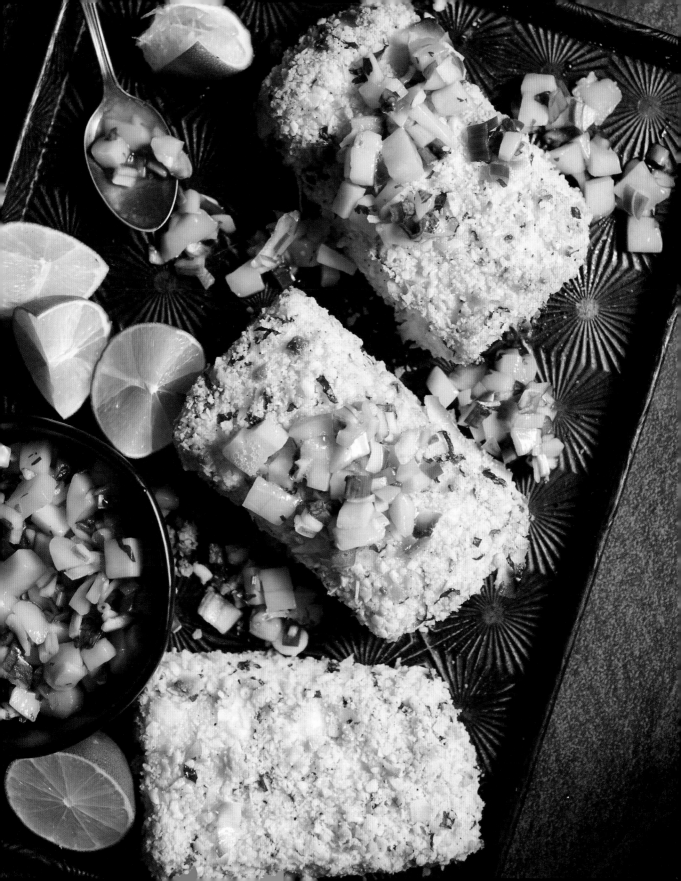

Serves:
6

Prep time:
20 minutes

Cook time:
45 minutes

I grew up on comforting oven-baked dishes, and tuna pasta bake was always one of my favourites. My husband says that even if this was the only recipe in the whole book, it would still sell. It's very easy to customize this dish by mixing up the vegetables or choosing any other ingredients you'd like to add.

Tuna Pasta Bake

125g (4½oz) gluten-free pasta shapes

60g (2oz) salted butter

1 celery stick, finely chopped

1 tbsp finely chopped onion

2 tbsp No. 1 All-Purpose Flour Blend (see p24)

½ tsp salt

¼ tsp freshly ground black pepper

500ml (16fl oz) whole milk

200g (7oz) coarsely grated mature Cheddar cheese

125g (4½oz) frozen peas, defrosted

2 x 140g cans of tuna in spring water, drained

50g (1¾oz) Home-Made Breadcrumbs (see p25) or shop-bought plain gluten-free breadcrumbs

1. Preheat the oven to 180°C (160°C fan/350°F/Gas 4). Bring a medium saucepan of salted water to the boil, and add the pasta. Cook the pasta for 3–5 minutes less than directed by the package instructions. Drain, and immediately rinse the pasta under cold water. Drain it again.

2. In a large saucepan, melt half the butter over a medium heat. Add the celery and onion and sauté until soft and translucent.

3. Add 15g (½oz) more butter to the saucepan, and stir until melted. Stir in the No. 1 All-Purpose Flour Blend, salt, and pepper. Stir constantly over a medium heat until smooth and bubbly.

4. Gradually stir in the milk and bring to the boil, constantly stirring. Once the milk begins to boil, stir for 1 minute more.

5. Stir in three-quarters of the Cheddar until melted and then remove from the heat. Fold in the drained pasta, peas, and tuna until well mixed.

6. Pour into a 2 litre (3½ pint) casserole dish and sprinkle the remaining Cheddar on top. Cover and cook for 25 minutes or until bubbly.

7. Meanwhile, prepare the crumb topping. In a small bowl, melt the remaining butter. Stir in the breadcrumbs.

8. After 25 minutes, uncover the casserole dish. Sprinkle the buttered breadcrumbs on top and cook, uncovered, for an additional 5 minutes. Let rest for 5 minutes, then serve.

Makes:
10

Prep time:
15 minutes

Cook time:
20 minutes

1 large egg

½ tsp salt

¼ tsp freshly ground black pepper

¼ tsp celery salt

¼ tsp paprika

3 tbsp mayonnaise

1 tsp lemon juice

1 tbsp Dijon mustard

1 tsp Worcestershire sauce (gluten-free)

1 tbsp chopped chives

1 tbsp chopped flat-leaf parsley

450g (1lb) fresh white crabmeat (defrosted, moisture squeezed out, and patted dry, if frozen)

100g (3½oz) crushed gluten-free crackers (see tip, right)

cooking spray, for coating

lemon wedges, to serve

For the cocktail sauce

60g (2oz) tomato ketchup

2 tsp horseradish sauce (gluten-free)

¼ tsp lemon juice

½ tsp light brown sugar

These crab cakes are prepared with gluten-free crackers and real crabmeat ("crab sticks" contain wheat), and then baked instead of fried. They are moist on the inside and crispy on the outside without any of the usual frying oil. Serve alongside home-made cocktail sauce and a lemon wedge for a great starter or main course.

Cracklin' Crab Cakes

1. Preheat the oven to 200°C (180°C fan/400°F/Gas 6) and line a baking tray with baking parchment.

2. In a large bowl, lightly beat the egg. Add the salt, pepper, celery salt, paprika, mayonnaise, lemon juice, Dijon mustard, Worcestershire sauce, chives, and parsley. Whisk until well combined.

3. Gently stir in the crabmeat, then the crushed crackers, until well combined.

4. Use your hands to form the mixture into patties. Be sure to squeeze it tightly, so the cakes will not fall apart when baked. Place on the prepared baking tray.

5. Lightly spray each cake with cooking spray and bake for 7 minutes. Flip the cakes, spray with cooking spray again, and bake for an additional 7 minutes.

6. Preheat the grill on its highest setting and grill both sides of the crab cakes for a couple of minutes to crisp up the outsides.

7. Meanwhile, make the cocktail sauce. In a small bowl, stir together the ketchup, horseradish, lemon juice, and brown sugar until well combined. Refrigerate until ready to use.

8. Serve the crab cakes as soon as they are ready, with lemon wedges and the home-made cocktail sauce.

Store it
Wrap each crab cake individually in cling film. Store in an airtight container in the freezer for up to 3 months.

Tip
You can use any gluten-free cracker, or you can also substitute breadcrumbs. To crush the crackers, place them in a resealable bag, press out the air, seal, and roll a rolling pin over the bag until the crackers are finely crushed.

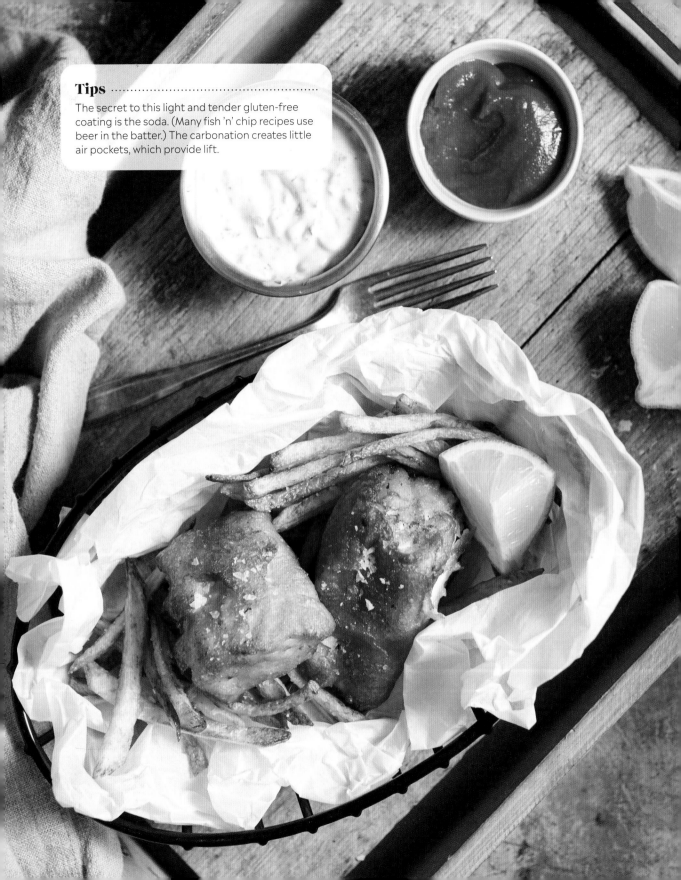

Tips

The secret to this light and tender gluten-free
coating is the soda. (Many fish 'n' chip recipes use
beer in the batter.) The carbonation creates little
air pockets, which provide lift.

Serves:
4

Prep time:
1½ hours, plus 1 hour to soak

Cook time:
30 minutes

Special equipment:
cooking thermometer

3 large Maris Piper
potatoes, peeled
and sliced into 5mm
(¼in) chips

1.5–3 litres (2¾–5¼ pints)
high smoke-point oil
(such as avocado oil),
for deep-frying

240g (8½oz) No. 1
All-Purpose Flour Blend
(see p24), plus extra
if needed

1 tsp garlic salt

1 tsp lemon pepper
seasoning

3 large egg whites

1½ tsp baking powder

½ tsp xanthan gum

1½ tsp salt, plus more
for seasoning

350–600ml (12–20fl oz)
fizzy lemon-lime drink
(such as Sprite or 7-Up)

680g (1½lb) skinless cod,
haddock, or halibut
fillets

For the tartare sauce

60g (2oz) mayonnaise

1½ tbsp sweet pickle relish

½ tsp dried parsley

1 tsp finely grated onion

salt and freshly ground
black pepper

Gluten-free fried foods are almost impossible to find when you are eating out. Living in Southern California, fish 'n' chips are on menus at restaurants all over town and they always smell so good! These gluten-free fish 'n' chips will rival any you would get in a restaurant.

Seaside Fish 'n' Chips

1. Soak the potato chips in cold water for at least 1 hour, or up to 24 hours. Drain, rinse well, and spread out the chips on kitchen paper to dry.

2. Once dry, pre-fry the potatoes. Fill a deep-fryer, heavy-based deep saucepan, or heavy flameproof casserole dish with oil about 7.5cm (3in) deep. Heat the oil to 160°C (325°F). (If the oil is not hot enough, the chips will be soggy.)

3. Working in batches so you don't overcrowd the pan, carefully add the potato to the hot oil. Fry for 3 minutes, drain, and spread on a kitchen paper-lined baking tray. (The potatoes will not be fully cooked yet.)

4. Prepare 3 shallow dishes. In the first, stir together 80g (2¾oz) of the No. 1 All-Purpose Flour Blend, the garlic salt, and lemon pepper seasoning. In the second, whisk the egg whites. In the third, whisk together the remaining 160g (5¾oz) No. 1 All-Purpose Flour Blend, baking powder, xanthan gum, and salt. Gradually whisk in the 350ml (12fl oz) of lemon-lime drink until smooth: it should be a runny batter. If it's too thick, gradually whisk in more fizzy drink 1 tablespoon at a time to reach the desired consistency, and if it's too thin, whisk in more flour 1 tablespoon at a time.

5. Increase the oil temperature to 190°C (375°F). Dredge the fish in the dry flour mixture, then in the egg whites, then in the batter, allowing excess to fall off.

6. Working in batches to avoid overcrowding, place the fish and a handful of pre-fried potatoes in the oil and cook for 5–7 minutes until golden brown.

7. Lift the fish and chips out of the oil with a slotted spoon and transfer to a kitchen paper-lined baking sheet or cooling rack. Sprinkle salt on the chips. Keep warm while you continue frying the rest of the fish and chips.

8. Meanwhile, to make the tartare sauce, in a small bowl, stir the mayonnaise, relish, parsley, onion, salt, and pepper. Refrigerate until ready to serve.

9. Serve the fish and chips as soon as they are all ready with the tartare sauce.

    Air Fryer Method: Preheat the air fryer to 200°C (400°F) to cook the chips for perfect crispiness. There's no need to soak or pre-fry the potatoes. (You cannot use an air fryer to cook the fish, as the batter is too runny.) Working in batches so you don't overcrowd the fryer basket, cook for 20–25 minutes, shaking every 5–8 minutes so the chips brown evenly.

Serves:
4–6

Prep time:
30 minutes

Cook time:
30 minutes

We love to prepare this easy recipe for midweek meals. The spiced mayonnaise mixed with the pico de gallo is what makes it so good. I will often serve the two sauces with beans and rice the next day for a tasty leftover dish. You could substitute chicken for the fish if you prefer, it will taste just as amazing!

Baja Fish Tacos

6 x 110–170g (4–6oz) fish fillets (halibut or any other mild white fish)

lemon pepper seasoning, to taste

garlic salt, to taste

½ green cabbage

8–10 corn tortillas

cooked rice, to serve

For the pico de gallo

5–6 plum tomatoes, finely chopped

3 tbsp chopped red onion

1 garlic clove, very finely chopped

1 tsp garlic salt

2 tbsp chopped coriander

freshly ground black pepper

For the spiced mayo

115g (4oz) mayonnaise

2 tbsp whole milk

1 tsp lemon juice

½ tsp garlic salt

½ tsp chipotle paste (optional)

For the black beans

1 tbsp avocado oil, or other vegetable oil

1 tbsp chopped onion

2 garlic cloves, very finely chopped

420g can of black beans

⅛ tsp chilli powder

¼ tsp ground cumin

¼ tsp dried oregano

½ tsp garlic salt

1. Preheat the barbecue for the fish (see tip, below), if using. Meanwhile, make the sauces and the beans.

2. For the pico de gallo, in a small bowl, stir together the tomatoes, red onion, garlic, garlic salt, coriander, and pepper. Adjust the seasonings to taste and refrigerate until ready to use.

3. To make the spiced mayo, in another small bowl, whisk together the mayonnaise, milk, lemon juice, garlic salt, and chipotle paste (if using), and refrigerate until ready to use.

4. For the beans, in a medium saucepan, heat the oil. Sauté the onion for about 5 minutes until tender and translucent. Add the garlic and cook for 1 minute. Stir in the black beans, chilli powder, cumin, oregano, and garlic salt, and bring to the boil. Reduce the heat to a simmer and cook for 5–10 minutes. Then, in a blender process about one-quarter of the contents of the saucepan until smooth. Mix back in with the beans and keep warm.

5. Preheat a griddle pan over a medium-high heat, if not using a barbecue. Season the fish with lemon pepper seasoning and garlic salt. Cook for 5–7 minutes on each side, until no longer opaque in the centre and it flakes easily with a fork.

6. While the fish is cooking, shred the cabbage and warm the tortillas in a dry frying pan over a medium heat.

7. Assemble the tacos. Layer the fish, cabbage, pico de gallo, and spiced mayo in the tortillas, and serve alongside the black beans and rice.

Tips

Make the pico de gallo and spiced mayo in the morning. The longer they sit and marinate, the more flavoursome they will be. Plus, dinner prep will be that much easier.

We prefer the flavour of barbecued fish here; however, fish fillets can be tricky on the barbecue because they often fall apart, stick, or fall through the grate. For the best success, you can either brush the grates with oil before placing the fish on the grill bars, or oil a sheet of aluminium foil and use it as a "pan" on the grill bars.

Serves:
6

Prep time:
1 hour

Cook time:
45 minutes

For the mash

1½ tsp salt

1.5kg (3lb 3oz) Maris Piper
    potatoes, peeled
    and cubed

75g (2½oz) salted butter

¼ tsp freshly ground
    black pepper

60ml (2fl oz) sour cream
    (optional; for extra
    creaminess)

For the filling

350-425g (12-15oz) raw
    chicken, cut into 2.5cm
    (1in) pieces

25g (scant 1oz) chopped
    onion

25g (scant 1oz) chopped
    celery

2 garlic cloves, very finely
    chopped

1 tsp salt

½ tsp freshly ground
    black pepper

360-480ml (12-16
    fl oz) chicken stock

150g (5½oz) carrot slices,
    5mm (¼in) thick

1 tsp dried thyme

1 tsp dried parsley

85g (3oz) No. 1 All-
    Purpose Flour Blend
    (see p24)

60g (2oz) frozen peas,
    defrosted

150g (5½oz) grated
    Cheddar cheese

I grew up on this chicken shepherd's pie. To this day, I still have never tried a traditional lamb shepherd's pie, and once you eat this version, you might never feel the need to go back, either! This recipe is full of comforting flavours.

Chicken Shepherd's Pie

1. Prepare the mash. Bring a large saucepan of water with 1 teaspoon of salt to the boil. Add the potatoes and cook for 18–20 minutes, or until tender.

2. Reserve 300ml (10fl oz) of the cooking water and then drain the potatoes. Place the potatoes in a large bowl. Use a potato masher to mash the potatoes.

3. Beat in the butter, the remaining ½ teaspoon salt, pepper, and sour cream (if using) with a wooden spoon. Now beat in up to 120ml (4fl oz) of the reserved cooking liquid, depending on the consistency you prefer, until smooth and fluffy. If it's too thick, add more of the reserved cooking liquid until you reach the desired consistency. Set aside.

4. Prepare the filling. Preheat the oven to 180°C (160°C fan/350°F/Gas 4). In a medium saucepan, evenly arrange the chicken. Add the onion, celery, garlic, salt, and pepper.

5. Pour in enough of the stock to just cover the chicken and vegetables, then bring to the boil, cover, and reduce the heat to low. Cook for 15 minutes.

6. Uncover the chicken, increase the heat to medium-high, and add the carrots, thyme, and parsley. Cook for 5 minutes.

7. In a small bowl, whisk the No. 1 All-Purpose Flour Blend with another 60ml (2fl oz) of the stock. Stir into the chicken mixture with the peas. Cook until thick and bubbly.

8. Pour the mixture into a 2.5 litre (4½ pint) baking dish. If the potatoes have become too thick from sitting, add the reserved cooking liquid 1 tablespoon at a time until smooth and easy to spread. Gently spread the mash evenly over the chicken mixture.

9. Sprinkle the Cheddar on top. Bake for 25–30 minutes or until heated through and bubbling. Let sit for 5 minutes before serving.

Tip ···

If the filling is too runny, the mash will have difficulty sitting on top of it and will sink. To prevent this, avoid using too much stock when cooking the chicken; use just enough to barely cover it and no more than suggested. If the filling still seems too watery toward the end of cooking, add more flour, 1 tablespoon at a time, until thick and bubbly.

Serves:
6 as a starter, or
3–4 as a main course

Prep time:
10 minutes

Cook time:
45 minutes

1 tsp garlic powder

1 tsp onion powder

1 tsp salt

½ tsp paprika

½ tsp freshly ground
black pepper

1.5–2kg (3lb 3oz–4½lb)
chicken wings, wing tips
discarded, halved
through the joints

flavourless vegetable oil,
for greasing

225g (8oz) salted butter,
melted (or less if you
prefer a hotter sauce),
plus extra for the tray

340g jar of gluten-free
hot sauce (such as
Frank's)

For the ranch dressing

115g (4oz) mayonnaise

120ml (4fl oz) sour cream

120ml (4fl oz) buttermilk

1½ tsp lemon juice

½ tsp garlic powder

2 tbsp chopped chives

3 tbsp chopped flat-leaf
parsley

½ tsp dried dill

½ tsp onion powder

½ tsp salt

¼ tsp freshly ground
black pepper

There is nothing better than a plate of spicy chicken wings and ranch dressing when bingeing on your favourite box set. My dad has been making these wings for every sporting event on television for years. They are so easy, have just the right amount of heat, and are sure to satisfy your guests. But have napkins ready: they are messy!

Pop's Chicken Wings
with Home-Made Ranch Dressing

1. Preheat the oven to 220°C (200°C fan/425°F/Gas 7). In a small bowl, stir together the garlic powder, onion powder, salt, paprika, and pepper.

2. In a large bowl, toss the spice blend with the chicken wings until they are evenly coated.

3. Grease a large baking tray or baking dish. Spread the wings out on the tray or dish and bake for 30–40 minutes or until browned.

4. In a small bowl, stir together all the ingredients for the ranch dressing and refrigerate until ready to serve.

5. Meanwhile, in a large bowl, whisk together the melted butter and hot sauce. Remove the wings from the oven and toss them with the hot sauce mixture.

6. Preheat the grill on its highest setting. Spread the wings back out onto the baking tray and grill for 1–2 minutes or until crispy.

7. Arrange the wings on a platter. Serve hot with any remaining hot sauce from the large bowl and the ranch dressing for dipping.

Air Fryer Method: An air fryer gets these wings extra crispy in a way the oven cannot. Prepare the wings as described in steps 1 and 2. Working in batches as needed, place the wings in the air fryer basket (do not overcrowd; wings shouldn't be touching) and spray all sides of the wings with cooking spray. Set the air fryer to 190°C (375°F), and cook for 25 minutes, shaking the basket halfway through cooking. Then increase the temperature to 200°C (400°F) and cook for an additional 5 minutes. Remove from the air fryer and toss immediately in the hot sauce mixture.

Tip ....
You can prepare the ranch dressing up to 2 days ahead, cover, and refrigerate, so the flavours can meld.

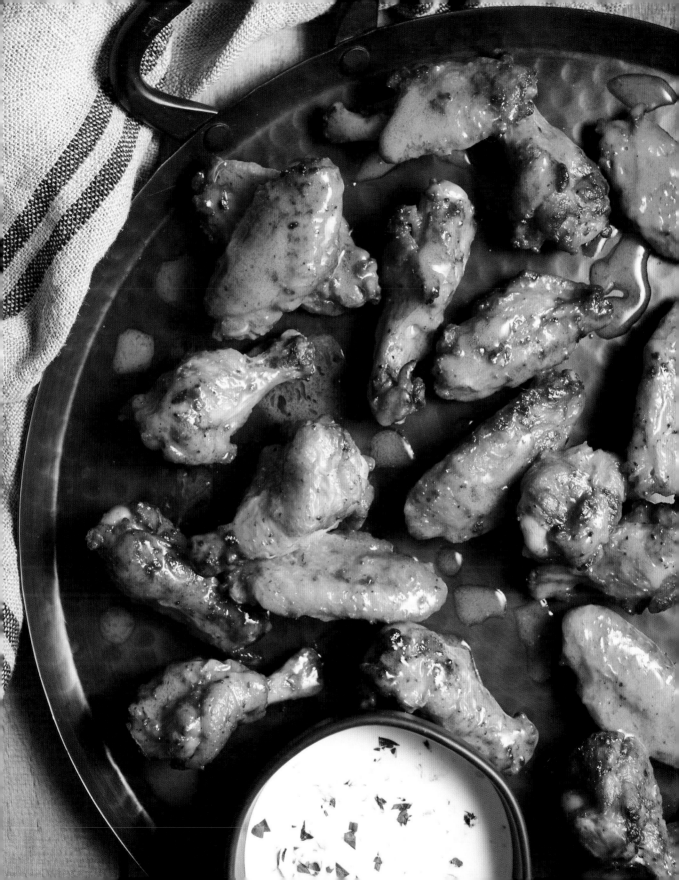

cooking spray, for greasing

3 large boneless, skinless chicken breasts, butterflied

80g (2¾oz) No. 1 All-Purpose Flour Blend (see p24)

1 tsp garlic salt

2 large eggs

100g (3½oz) Home-Made Breadcrumbs (see p25) or shop-bought plain gluten-free breadcrumbs

1 tsp dried basil

1 tsp dried oregano

1 tsp dried parsley

½ tsp salt

¼ tsp freshly ground black pepper

2 tbsp avocado oil, or other vegetable oil, plus extra if needed

900g-1.1kg (2-2½lb) Mum's Famous Meat Sauce (see p82), or your favourite meaty pasta sauce

35g (1¼oz) grated Parmesan cheese, for topping, or to taste

340g (12oz) block of mozzarella cheese, cut into 12 slices

We enjoy eating this alongside steamed broccoli, but it is also very good served on top of gluten-free spaghetti. The home-made Mum's Famous Meat Sauce (see p82) is what makes this dish so special, but you can substitute any other meaty pasta sauce.

Chicken Parmesan

1. Preheat the oven to 190°C (170°C fan/375°F/Gas 5) and lightly grease a large baking tray with cooking spray.

2. One at a time, place the butterflied chicken breasts between 2 sheets of baking parchment or cling film and gently pound out until about 5mm (¼in) thick.

3. Prepare 3 shallow dishes. In the first, stir together the No. 1 All-Purpose Flour Blend and garlic salt. In the second, beat the eggs. In the third, stir together the breadcrumbs, basil, oregano, parsley, salt, and pepper.

4. In a large frying pan, heat the oil over a medium-high heat. Dredge each chicken breast in the No. 1 All-Purpose Flour Blend, then the eggs, letting excess drip off, and then coat thoroughly on all sides in the breadcrumb mixture, pressing the chicken in lightly so the crumbs stick.

5. Fry for 3–4 minutes on each side or until golden brown, adding more oil if the pan becomes too dry. Transfer the chicken breasts to the prepared baking tray.

6. Top each piece of chicken with an equal amount of Mum's Famous Meat Sauce, sprinkle with Parmesan, then cover each with 2 slices of mozzarella.

7. Bake for 20 minutes, or until the sauce is bubbly and the cheese is melted and golden brown. Serve immediately.

Serves:
6

Prep time:
15 minutes

Cook time:
40 minutes

680g (1½lb) broccoli
    florets, cut into
    bite-sized pieces

420g (15oz) cooked
    chicken breasts, cubed

680g (1½lb) condensed
    gluten-free cream of
    chicken soup (available
    online, or in health food
    shops, see tip, below)

225g (8oz) mayonnaise

1 tsp lemon juice

110g (4oz) Cheddar
    cheese, grated

Any time I ask my husband what he wants for dinner, the answer is chicken divan, his all-time favourite dish. He loves anything with a sauce, and this recipe, using only three ingredients, creates a creamy, flavoursome sauce that the broccoli and chicken soak right up.

Divine Chicken Divan

1. Preheat the oven to 180°C (160°C fan/350°F/Gas 4). Put the broccoli florets in a large saucepan, and cover with about 5cm (2in) water. Cover and cook over a high heat for 4–6 minutes depending on the desired tenderness.

2. Drain the broccoli and spread out evenly in a 33 x 23cm (13 x 9in) baking dish. Arrange the cooked chicken cubes evenly over the broccoli.

3. In a medium bowl, stir together the soup, mayonnaise, and lemon juice until well combined. Pour the soup mixture on top of the chicken and broccoli and spread out evenly, being sure to cover every piece so that they do not dry out in the oven.

4. Sprinkle the Cheddar evenly over the top. Bake for 30–35 minutes or until bubbly. Let rest for 5–10 minutes before serving.

Tip ....

You can prep this meal up to 24 hours ahead of baking. Cover the fully prepared dish and refrigerate until ready to bake.

This recipe was developed using condensed chicken soup. If you can only find thinner varieties of chicken soup, you may need to thicken the sauce at the end of cooking time. To do this, add No. 1 All-Purpose Flour Blend (see p24), 1 tbsp at a time, and return the sauce to a gentle simmer after each addition until it thickens to your liking. Taste to see if you also need more salt, then serve.

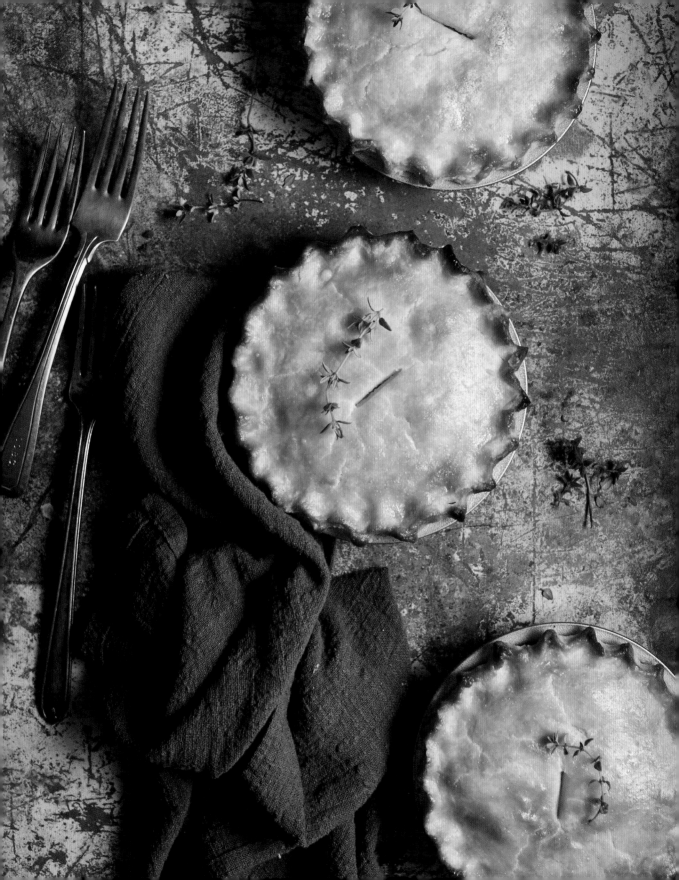

Makes:
1 x 23cm (9in) pie
or 8–10 mini pies

Prep time:
40 minutes

Cook time:
55 minutes

2 raw Buttery Pastry discs
(see p138)

150g (5½oz) Maris Piper
potatoes, peeled and
chopped

45g (1½oz) sliced carrots

2 tsp salt

115g (4oz) salted butter

50g (1¾oz) chopped
onion

50g (1¾oz) chopped
celery

2 garlic cloves, very finely
chopped

¼ tsp freshly ground
black pepper

¼ tsp garlic powder

¼ tsp onion powder

80g (2¾oz) No. 1
All-Purpose Flour Blend
(see p24)

350ml (12fl oz) chicken
stock

120ml (4fl oz) dry white
wine, or 60ml (2fl oz)
each white wine vinegar
and water

180ml (6fl oz) whole milk

300g (10oz) cooked
chicken, cubed

70g (2½oz) frozen peas,
defrosted

1½ tsp dried parsley

1 tsp dried thyme

1 large egg

1 tbsp water

I have been told, "This is the best chicken pot pie I have ever had!" It has a flaky, buttery crust, and a rich, creamy filling of chicken and vegetables. I love to make these as individual servings so everyone can have their own pie, or you can stock the freezer and have them ready for lunches and dinners.

World's Best Chicken Pot Pie

1. Roll out half the pastry and use it to line a 23cm (9in) deep pie dish. Freeze until ready to use. Roll out the other half into a circle for a lid and refrigerate, pulling it out of the refrigerator 5 minutes before you need it. Preheat the oven to 220°C (200°C fan/425°F/Gas 7).

2. Put the potatoes, carrots, and ½ tsp salt in a small saucepan. Add water to just cover the vegetables. Bring to the boil over a high heat, then reduce the heat to low, cover, and cook for 8 minutes. Strain and set aside.

3. In a large frying pan, heat the butter over a medium-high heat. Add the onion and celery and sauté until tender. Add the garlic and cook for 1 minute more. Add the pepper, 1½ tsp salt, garlic and onion powders, and No. 1 All-Purpose Flour Blend, and stir until combined. Gradually stir in the stock, wine, and milk. Cook, stirring constantly, until thick and bubbly.

4. Stir in the chicken, peas, parsley, thyme, and potato mixture. Taste and adjust the seasoning as desired. Remove from the heat.

5. Remove the pie crust base from the freezer and fill with the chicken mixture. Place the refrigerated top crust over the filling and seal the edges.

6. In a small bowl, lightly beat together the egg and water. Brush the top of the pie with the egg wash, and then cut 1 or 2 slits in the crust.

7. Bake for 35–40 minutes or until the crust is lightly browned. Check the pie halfway through cooking; if the edges are getting too brown, cover them with foil. Let the pie rest for 15 minutes before serving.

Mini Pies: Using 2 raw Buttery Pastry discs and 10cm (4in) pie dishes, this recipe will make 8–10 mini pies. (You will not place a bottom crust into the tins.)

In step 1, cut the rolled-out pie crusts into circles to fit on top of your dishes, then refrigerate. (You don't need to freeze any crust.) In step 5, fill each pan almost to the top with the filling; be sure to seal the top crust to the dishes so the filling does not bubble out.

Serves:
6

Prep time:
20 minutes, plus up to
12 hours to marinate

Cook time:
1 hour 10 minutes

Special equipment:
probe thermometer

1.5–1.6kg (3lb 3oz–3½lb)
  chicken thighs and
  drumsticks, bone-in and
  skin-on, trimmed of
  excess skin
450ml (15fl oz) buttermilk
360g (13oz) No. 1
  All-Purpose Flour Blend
  (see p24)
¾ tsp xanthan gum
3 tsp paprika
3 tsp salt
¾ tsp freshly ground
  black pepper
¾ tsp garlic powder
¾ tsp onion powder
40g (1½oz) freshly grated
  Parmesan cheese
115g (4oz) salted butter

This chicken contains all the flavour and crispiness of fried chicken without actually being fried. The high heat of the oven gets the skin nice and crispy, and the gluten-free flour coating is full of spices and flavour. My whole family loves fried chicken, and this is much better than a bucket from the takeaway.

Oven "Fried" Chicken

1. Divide the chicken pieces evenly between two resealable plastic bags. Add half the buttermilk to each bag. Place in the refrigerator, making sure all the chicken pieces are coated. Marinate all day, or overnight.

2. Preheat the oven to 220°C (200°C fan/425°F/Gas 7). In a small bowl, stir together the No. 1 All-Purpose Flour Blend, xanthan gum, paprika, salt, pepper, garlic powder, onion powder, and Parmesan until well combined.

3. Pour the flour mixture into a separate large resealable bag. One piece at a time, add the chicken pieces to the bag, seal, and shake until well coated. Place the coated chicken pieces on a wire rack. Repeat until all the pieces have been coated. Repeat with all the chicken pieces for a second coat. Discard the buttermilk.

4. Place the butter in a large baking tray and melt in the oven. Place the chicken skin side down in the tray and bake for 40 minutes.

5. Very carefully, so you don't lose any of the coating, flip the chicken with a spatula and fork (see tip, below) and bake for an additional 20–30 minutes or until the internal temperature reaches 74°C (165°F) and the skin is very crispy. Serve immediately.

    Air Fryer Method: Follow the instructions to the end of step 3. Preheat the air fryer to 180°C (350°F). Spray the skin side of the chicken with cooking oil. Place the chicken pieces skin side down into the air fryer basket. Spray the other side with cooking oil. Air fry for 15 minutes. Flip the chicken and spray with more oil if the skin is looking dry, or if any flour has not been coated with oil. Cook for an additional 10–12 minutes or until the internal temperature reaches 74°C (165°F).

Tip

The coating falls off very easily when flipping the chicken. Use a spatula to scrape under the chicken when flipping, and use a fork to help gently guide it onto its other side. Using tongs is a little too rough and will scrape the coating off. A fish slice also works.

Chicken piccata always seems like a fancy dish you would only eat in restaurants, but it is actually very easy to make using very few ingredients. Serve this dish to your family, and they will think they just sat down at an elegant Italian restaurant.

Chicken Piccata

680g (1½lb) boneless, skinless chicken breasts, butterflied

160g (5¾oz) No. 1 All-Purpose Flour Blend (see p24)

½ tsp garlic salt

¼ tsp freshly ground black pepper, plus more for seasoning

4 tbsp freshly grated Parmesan cheese

2 tbsp avocado oil, or other vegetable oil

60g (2oz) salted butter

1 tsp salt

60ml (2fl oz) chicken stock

90ml (3fl oz) white wine

3 tbsp lemon juice

40g (1½oz) capers in brine

1½ tsp chopped flat-leaf parsley

1. Preheat a small dish in the oven at 140°C (120°C fan/275°F/Gas 1) to keep the chicken warm once cooked. One at a time, place the chicken breasts between 2 sheets of baking parchment or cling film and gently pound out until about 5mm (¼in) thick.

2. In a shallow dish, stir together the No. 1 All-Purpose Flour Blend, garlic salt, ¼ teaspoon pepper, and Parmesan.

3. In a large frying pan, heat the avocado oil over a medium-high heat. Melt half the butter in the oil.

4. Salt and pepper both sides of each chicken breast, and then dredge each piece in the flour mixture. Fry each piece of flour-coated chicken in the butter and oil for 4–5 minutes on each side, or until cooked all the way through and golden brown. (You may have to cook them in batches.) Transfer each piece of cooked chicken to the dish in the oven.

5. In the same pan used to fry the chicken, add the stock, wine, lemon juice, and capers, and use them to deglaze the pan, stirring to remove any tasty morsels stuck to the pan. Reduce the heat to medium and reduce the liquid by half.

6. Whisk in the remaining butter and the parsley. Stir until the butter is melted. Return the chicken to the pan over a medium heat and slightly reduce the sauce. Serve immediately.

Tip ....

Prepare some of this dish ahead of time. Flatten the chicken up to 1 day in advance, storing it in the refrigerator separated by pieces of baking parchment in a resealable bag. You can also mix together the flour, seasonings, and Parmesan and store in the refrigerator until ready to use.

Serves:
3–4

Prep time:
15 minutes, plus
30 minutes to chill

Cook time:
None

115g (4oz) mayonnaise

1 tsp Dijon mustard

¼ tsp dried dill

1 tbsp finely chopped red onion

2 tbsp finely chopped celery

2–3 tbsp finely chopped dill gherkins

300g (10oz) cooked chicken, chopped

1 small carrot, grated

salt and freshly ground black pepper

Easy White Sandwich Bread (see p113) or shop-bought gluten-free bread; lettuce; or gluten-free crackers and celery sticks, to serve

The gherkins give this chicken salad a bit of sour flavour that is perfectly balanced by the sweetness in the carrots. I started putting the carrots in this salad just for a little additional nutrition, but we loved the flavour so much that now it's a standard ingredient.

Chicken Salad

1. In a medium bowl, stir together the mayonnaise, mustard, dill, onion, and celery.

2. Gently stir in the gherkins and chicken. Fold in the grated carrot and season with salt and pepper to taste.

3. Chill for at least 30 minutes. Serve on slices of bread, on a bed of lettuce, or with crackers and celery sticks for scooping.

Tip ....

This chicken salad is great at a buffet. You can serve it in a bowl with crackers, or carrot and celery sticks, to use for dipping. You can also put small amounts into bite-sized radicchio lettuce "cups".

Serves:
4

Prep time:
15 minutes

Cook time:
40 minutes

These white chicken enchiladas are smothered in a simple, rich, creamy sauce and topped with cheese. I can honestly say this was my favourite meal growing up, and with a great gluten-free flour tortilla, this recipe is pretty close to the dish of my memories.

Creamy White Chicken Enchiladas

vegetable oil, for greasing

340g (12oz) condensed gluten-free cream of chicken soup (available online, or in specialist shops)

½ onion, chopped

100g can or jar of green chillies, chopped

240ml (8fl oz) sour cream

225g (8oz) Monterey Jack cheese, or mild Cheddar, grated

350g (12oz) cooked chicken, cubed or shredded

8 Flour Tortillas (see p117) or shop-bought gluten-free flour tortillas

1. Preheat the oven to 180°C (160°C fan/350°F/Gas 4) and lightly grease a 33 x 23cm (13 x 9in) baking dish. In a medium bowl, mix the cream of chicken soup, onion, chillies, sour cream, and half the cheese.

2. In a separate large bowl, stir together the chicken with half the sauce.

3. Place one-eighth of the chicken mixture on each tortilla, roll, and arrange seam side down in the prepared baking dish.

4. Pour the remaining cream sauce over the enchiladas, and spread out evenly. Sprinkle the remaining cheese on top.

5. Bake for 30–40 minutes or until hot and bubbly. Let rest for 5–10 minutes before serving.

Tip ....
Serve with sour cream and your favourite salsa or hot sauce. Salsa verde is excellent with these enchiladas.

Pork & Beef Mains

We go for lunch at my mum and dad's house almost every Sunday, and this dish is a staple. As I've mentioned, my family loves anything with sauce on it! Plus, with five grandsons who love to eat, this is one recipe that is easy to make in bulk. Serve with mashed potatoes, rice, noodles, asparagus, or green beans.

Pork Chops
with Mushroom Gravy

45g (1½oz) salted butter

10–12 thin-cut boneless pork chops (or 5–6 thick boneless pork chops, butterflied)

salt and freshly ground black pepper

1 small onion, halved and finely sliced

225g (8oz) sliced mushrooms

680g (1½lb) condensed gluten-free cream of mushroom soup (available online, or in health food shops, see tip, below)

1. In a large, deep frying pan or sauté pan, melt 30g (1oz) of the butter over a medium-high heat.

2. Season both sides of the pork chops with salt and pepper. Brown in the melted butter for 2–3 minutes per side. Remove the pork chops and set aside.

3. Melt the remaining butter in the pan and add the onion and mushrooms. Cook for 6–8 minutes or until tender. Stir in the cream of mushroom soup.

4. Return the pork chops to the pan. Bring to a simmer, then reduce the heat to low, cover, and cook for 45–60 minutes, stirring occasionally, until the pork chops are tender. Serve immediately.

Tip ....

Slowly cooking these chops over a very low heat is what makes them so tender. Don't rush the process.

This recipe was developed using condensed gluten-free mushroom soup. If you can only find thinner varieties of gluten-free mushroom soup, you may need to thicken the sauce at the end of cooking time. To do this, add No. 1 All-Purpose Flour Blend (see p24), 1 tbsp at a time, and return the sauce to a gentle simmer after each addition until it thickens to your liking. Taste to see if you also need more salt, then serve.

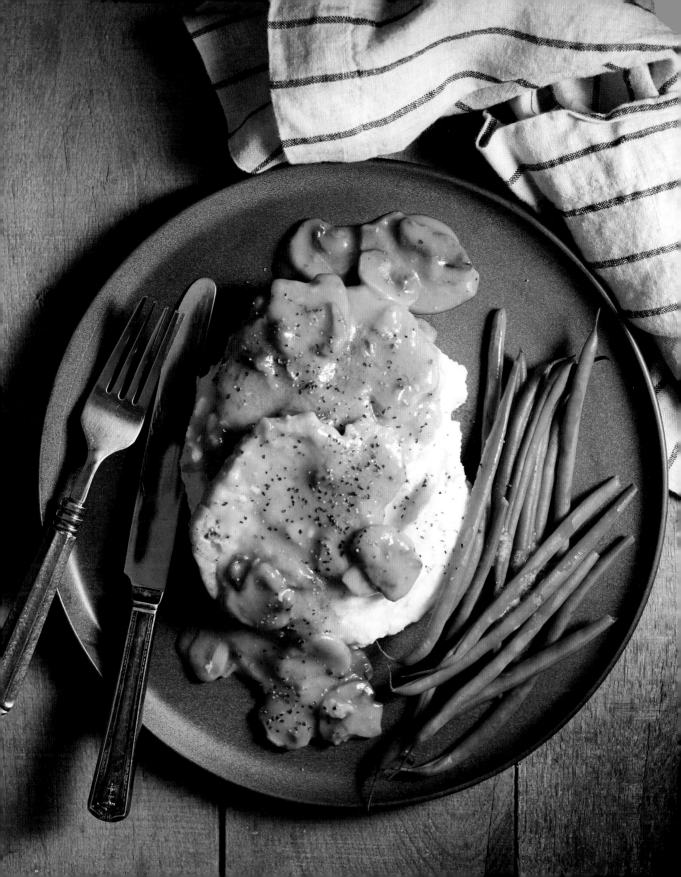

Serves:
6

Prep time:
10 minutes

Cook time:
45 minutes

Pork chops can be tricky and often turn out dry because they are a relatively quick-cooking, lean meat. However, when you cook chops slowly over a low heat and smother them in this light and creamy sauce, there is nothing dry about them. This recipe is great served alongside rice and roasted asparagus.

Heavenly Dijon Pork Chops

15g (½oz) salted butter

1 tbsp avocado oil, or other vegetable oil

6 pork chops (boneless or bone-in)

salt and freshly ground black pepper

40g (1¼oz) chopped shallots

120ml (4fl oz) dry white wine

180ml (6fl oz) chicken stock

1 tbsp No. 1 All-Purpose Flour Blend (see p24)

120ml (4fl oz) double cream

2 tsp Dijon mustard

1 tbsp chopped flat-leaf parsley

1. In a large deep frying pan, melt the butter and the oil over a medium-high heat. Season the chops with salt and pepper on both sides. Brown for 2–3 minutes on each side.

2. Remove the chops to a plate and pour off all but 1 tablespoon of the fat from the pan. Add the shallots and cook until softened, about 2 minutes.

3. Add the wine and deglaze the pan, scraping it with a wooden spoon to get all those tasty bits into the sauce, and bring to the boil. Stir in the stock and return the chops to the pan.

4. Bring the sauce to a simmer, reduce the heat to medium-low, cover, and cook until the pork chops are tender, about 20 minutes. Remove the pork chops to a serving dish. Cover to keep warm.

5. Increase the heat to medium-high and boil the juices in the pan until reduced by half. Whisk in the No. 1 All-Purpose Flour Blend. Whisk in the cream and mustard and boil for 2 more minutes, or until the sauce has thickened. Stir in the parsley and remove from the heat.

6. Taste the sauce and adjust the seasoning with salt and pepper. Pour it over the pork chops and serve immediately.

If you're in need of a super-easy no-prep meal, then here you go! With only two ingredients, this Mexican-style pork has as much flavour as if you had spent all day cooking. It's also very versatile: use it for tacos with shredded lettuce, sour cream, chopped red onions, coriander, and grated cheese, or serve it over rice with black beans.

Easy Slow-Cooker Salsa Verde Pork

1.35–1.8kg (3–4lb)
   boneless pork roast

1–2 x 450g jars salsa verde
   Mexican tomatillo sauce
   (such as Frontera,
   available online or in
   American and Mexican
   specialist shops)

1. Cut the pork roast into 3–4 large chunks and place it in a slow-cooker. Add the salsa verde: the more salsa you use, the saucier the pork will be in the end. One jar mostly just flavours the pork, while both will create a verde sauce for the pork to soak in.

2. Cook on low for 8 hours. After the cooking is complete, shred the pork with 2 forks. Stir until the meat is well combined with the salsa and juices, then serve immediately.

Store it
Store in an airtight container in the freezer for up to 3 months. Defrost in the refrigerator overnight or slowly reheat in a saucepan over a gentle heat.

Tip
If you want even more flavour, season the pork with salt and freshly ground black pepper and brown in oil for 5–10 minutes before tipping it into the slow-cooker with the salsa verde.

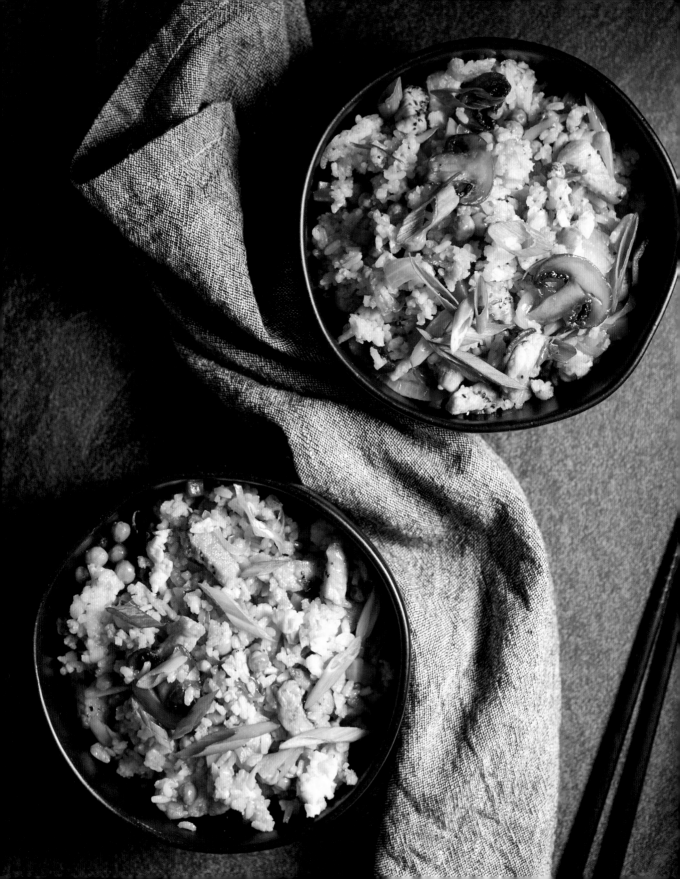

Serves:
4 for a main or
6–8 as a side

Prep time:
15 minutes

Cook time:
25 minutes

3 thin-cut boneless
   pork chops

½ tsp salt

¼ tsp freshly ground
   black pepper

3 tbsp avocado oil, or
   other vegetable oil

½ tsp toasted sesame oil

½ medium onion, halved
   and finely sliced

4 spring onions, cut on
   the diagonal, plus more
   to serve

60g (2oz) carrots, finely
   chopped

35g (1¼oz) mushrooms,
   sliced

1 tsp grated fresh root
   ginger

2 tbsp tamari, or coconut
   aminos

1.2kg (2¾lb) cold cooked
   long-grain rice (such as
   jasmine or brown rice)

100g (3½oz) frozen peas,
   defrosted

3 large eggs, lightly
   beaten

My dad often makes too much rice for an evening meal, leaving enough cooked rice to stir-fry this for lunch the next day. Chinese food has always been one of my favourites, but it's rare to find a Chinese restaurant that serves gluten-free food. This recipe uses tamari (a gluten-free soy sauce) or coconut aminos, making it wheat-free.

Papa Motte's Pork Fried Rice

1. Cut the pork chops into 2.5cm (1in) long slices and toss with the salt and pepper. In a large wok or large non-stick frying pan, heat 2 tablespoons of the avocado oil over a medium-high heat. Add the pork pieces and sauté until cooked all the way through and no longer pink in the middle. Remove from the pan and set aside.

2. Add the sesame oil to the same pan with the onion, spring onions, carrots, mushrooms, and ginger. Cook until tender-crisp and slightly chewy, about 5 minutes. Add the tamari and stir until spread well throughout. Remove the vegetables from the pan and set aside.

3. Add the remaining 1 tablespoon of avocado oil to the pan. Add the rice, increase the heat to high, and cook until slightly browned, stirring constantly.

4. Reduce the heat to medium, return the stir-fried vegetables and pork, and add the peas. Cook, stirring constantly, for 5 minutes.

5. Create a well in the middle of the rice mixture so that the pan is exposed. Pour the beaten eggs into the well and cook. Once cooked through, break up into pieces and stir through the rice mixture. Scatter with spring onions and serve immediately.

Store it
Store leftovers in an airtight container in the refrigerator for up to 5 days, or freeze individual portions in airtight containers for up to 3 months. Reheat in the microwave, or over a high heat, until piping hot throughout.

Tip
Day-old rice that has been in the refrigerator works really well for this recipe because the rice will fry up better if it is cold and a little dried out.

Serves:
6

Prep time:
10 minutes, plus 30 minutes to marinate

Cook time:
20 minutes

Special equipment:
probe thermometer

120ml (4fl oz) tamari, or coconut aminos
120ml (4fl oz) rice wine vinegar (gluten-free)
2 tbsp toasted sesame oil
2 tbsp raw honey
1 tsp grated fresh root ginger
2 garlic cloves, grated
½ tsp lemon pepper seasoning
1 large or 2 small pork tenderloins, about 1.5kg (3lb 3oz) in total

I have adapted this pork tenderloin recipe from my mother-in-law to be gluten-free. It is so luscious, full of flavour and easy to make. This tenderloin is cooked on the barbecue and makes a great meal for those hot days when you don't want to turn on your oven. I love serving it alongside rice and vegetables.

Linda's Barbecued Pork Tenderloin

1. In a small bowl, whisk together the tamari, rice wine vinegar, sesame oil, honey, ginger, garlic, and lemon pepper seasoning until well combined.

2. Pour the sauce into a large resealable bag. Add the pork and marinate for 30 minutes at room temperature. Preheat the barbecue to a medium heat, about 180°C (350°F).

3. Place the pork on the hot barbecue and discard the marinade. Grill for 14–16 minutes, turning every 3–4 minutes, until the internal temperature reaches at least 65°C (149°F) and the meat is cooked through but still moist, or a few minutes longer for well done.

4. Wrap the pork in foil and let it rest for 5 minutes. Carve on the diagonal, place on a serving dish, and pour any juices collected in the foil over the pork. Serve immediately.

Beef, mushrooms, cream sauce, and pasta come together in this classic dish that will soon become a regular on your table. The beef is slowly cooked in a rich, creamy sauce, giving it tons of flavour and making it super-moist and tender. My husband loves anything with a good sauce, and this has become one of his favourites.

Classic Beef Stroganoff

250–340g (9–12oz) gluten-free pasta (I like tagliatelle, or brown rice fusilli by Doves Farm)

1 tbsp avocado oil, or other vegetable oil

675g (1½lb) beef sirloin, cut into 2.5 x 1cm (1 x ½in) pieces

½ tsp salt, plus extra for seasoning

¼ tsp freshly ground black pepper, plus extra for seasoning

60g (2oz) salted butter

1 onion, halved and finely sliced

225g (8oz) sliced white mushrooms

480ml (16fl oz) beef stock

½ tsp dried thyme

2 tsp Worcestershire sauce (gluten-free)

40g (1¼oz) No. 1 All-Purpose Flour Blend (see p24)

1 tsp Dijon mustard

240ml (8fl oz) sour cream

1 tbsp chopped flat-leaf parsley

paprika, to serve

1. In a medium saucepan, cook the pasta according to the package instructions. Rinse immediately under cold water. Set aside.

2. In a large deep sauté pan, heat the oil over a medium-high heat. Season the beef with salt and pepper. Brown the beef in the hot oil for 2–3 minutes. Remove the meat from the pan.

3. Add the butter to the meat juices in the pan and melt. Add the onion and mushrooms. Cook just until soft, about 5 minutes.

4. Stir in half the beef stock, the measured salt and pepper, the thyme, and Worcestershire sauce. Return the meat to the pan and stir. Bring to the boil, reduce the heat, cover, and simmer for 15 minutes.

5. In a small bowl, whisk the No. 1 All-Purpose Flour Blend, mustard, and the remaining stock. Stir into the beef mixture. Bring to the boil and stir constantly for 1 minute.

6. Reduce the heat to low and stir in the sour cream and parsley. Cook until heated through, but do not boil. Taste and adjust the seasoning with more salt and pepper to taste. Sprinkle some paprika on top and serve immediately over the cooked pasta.

This recipe came about when we had leftover steak, but I didn't want to just eat a plain slice of cold meat. I absolutely love horseradish, so the creamy sauce in this recipe is heavenly to me. You can use leftover meat to make these sandwiches, or you can buy fresh and barbecue or griddle it as directed. The flavour combination is unbelievable.

Steak Sandwiches
with Horseradish Cream Sauce

30g (1oz) salted butter

1 tbsp avocado oil, or other vegetable oil

1 onion, sliced

450g (1lb) flank steak (bavette), sirloin, or your favourite cut of beef

salt and freshly ground black pepper

Easy White Sandwich Bread (see p113) or store-bought gluten-free bread or rolls, halved (see tip, below)

4-8 slices of medium strength cheese, ideally Munster or provolone

For the sauce

75g (2½oz) mayonnaise

1 tsp wholegrain mustard

5 tsp shop-bought horseradish sauce (gluten-free)

1. Preheat a barbecue, or place a griddle pan over a medium-high heat. In a medium frying pan over a medium-high heat, heat the butter and oil. Add the sliced onion to the frying pan and cook until very soft and slightly caramelized, about 15 minutes.

2. Meanwhile, season the meat with salt and pepper and barbecue or griddle until the desired doneness is reached, about 8 minutes per side for medium. Finely slice the cooked meat.

3. Preheat the grill on its highest setting. Lightly warm up or toast the bread or rolls. Spread the horseradish cream sauce on each slice of bread, or on the cut sides of each roll. Set the top slices of bread or rolls aside. Top the bottom slices of bread or rolls with meat, onion, and finally the sliced cheese. Place the bottom piece with the meat, onion, and cheese a few inches under the grill and cook until the cheese melts.

4. Place the top piece of bread or rolls on each sandwich. Serve them with more horseradish cream sauce on the side.

    Horseradish Cream Sauce: In a small bowl, stir together the mayonnaise, mustard, and horseradish. Refrigerate until ready to use.

Tip ....
I like to use gluten-free hot dog rolls when making these sandwiches.

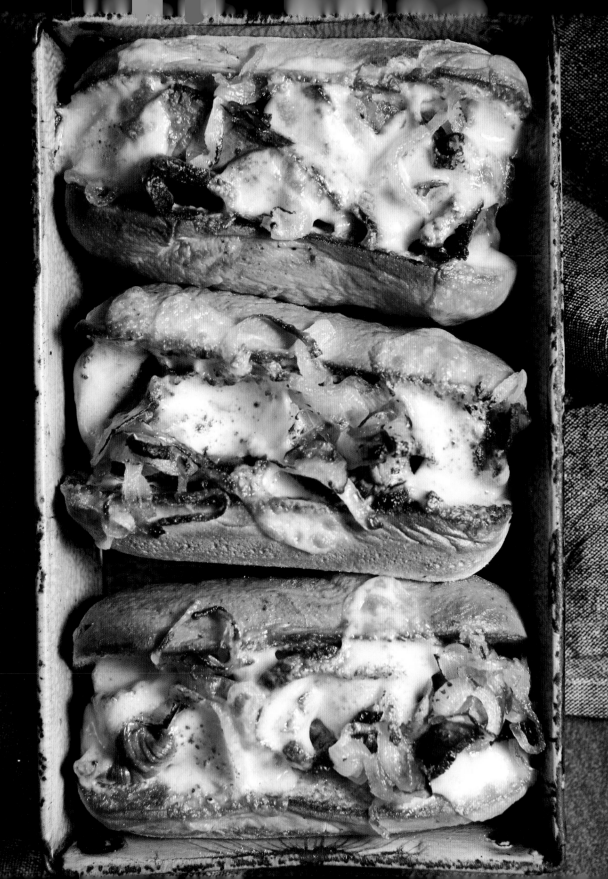

Serves:
8–10 (makes about 4.75 litres (8¼ pints)

Prep time:
20 minutes

Cook time:
2½ hours

2 tbsp avocado oil, or other vegetable oil

2 mild green chillies, ideally Anaheim or poblano

1 onion, chopped

2 garlic cloves, grated

1 tsp salt, plus extra for seasoning

½ tsp freshly ground black pepper, plus extra for seasoning

900g (2lb) chuck steak, or other stewing steak, cut into bite-sized pieces

400g can chopped tomatoes

480ml (16fl oz) beef stock

1 tsp chilli powder

1 tsp ground cumin

900g (2lb) minced beef

2 x 400g cans pinto beans, drained and unrinsed

400g can kidney beans, drained and rinsed

2 x 400g cans chilli beans (beans in mild chilli sauce)

sour cream, grated cheese, and tortilla chips (optional), to serve

My dad's chilli, or "Papa's Chilli" as it's known in our house, is the best chilli around. It's amazing on top of baked potatoes, with chips, tortilla chips, or just straight out of a bowl. It is so meaty and hearty: the perfect meal for a chilly day.

Papa's Meaty Chilli

1. In a very large saucepan or heavy flameproof casserole dish, heat the oil over a medium-high heat. While the oil is heating, slice the chillies in half, discard the seeds, and finely chop. Add the chillies and onion to the pot, and sauté for 5 minutes, or until soft and translucent. Add the garlic, salt, and pepper, and cook for 30 seconds more.

2. Season the steak with salt and pepper and add to the pan. Cook just until browned on all sides, stirring often.

3. Stir in the chopped tomatoes with their juices, beef stock, chilli powder, and cumin. Bring just to the boil, then reduce the heat to low, cover, and simmer for about 1 hour, or until the steak is tender.

4. Meanwhile, in a medium sauté pan, cook the minced beef over a medium heat until no longer pink, breaking it up into little pieces.

5. Add the minced beef to the casserole dish, along with the pinto beans, kidney beans, and chilli beans. Stir to combine and simmer for an additional 1 hour. Season with salt and pepper to taste. Serve immediately with the desired toppings.

Slow-Cooker Method: First follow steps 1 and 2 to sauté the chillies, onion, garlic, and steak in a large frying pan. Add the mixture to a slow-cooker, and brown the minced beef in the same frying pan. Then add all the ingredients to the slow-cooker. Cook on low for 6–8 hours or on high for 3–4 hours.

Store it
Store in an airtight container in the refrigerator for up to 5 days, or in the freezer for up to 6 months.

Tip
To make this red meat-free, substitute bite-sized pieces of chicken breast for the steak, minced turkey for the minced beef, and chicken stock for the beef stock.

Serves:
4

Prep time:
10 minutes

Cook time:
2 hours 20 minutes

This recipe came from my husband's grandma Joy and has been served at many family gatherings. We love to eat it with mashed potatoes. I have adapted this recipe to taste as close to the original version as possible. Do not rush the cooking time, as the low and slow cooking is what makes the meat so tender.

Grandma Joy's Swiss Steak

120g (4½oz) No. 1 All-Purpose Flour Blend (see p24)

1 tsp salt

4 tbsp avocado oil, or other vegetable oil

900g (2lb) beef silverside, cut into 4–6 steaks

1 onion, halved and finely sliced

750ml (1¼ pints) chicken stock

1½ tsp celery salt

⅛ tsp freshly ground black pepper

340g (12oz) condensed gluten-free cream of mushroom soup (available online, or in health food shops, see tip, below)

120ml (4fl oz) double cream

1. Preheat the oven to 150°C (130°C fan/300°F/Gas 2). In a medium shallow dish, stir together 65g (2¼oz) of the No. 1 All-Purpose Flour Blend and ½ teaspoon of the salt.

2. In a large non-stick frying pan, heat 3 tablespoons of the oil over a medium-high heat.

3. Dredge each piece of meat in the seasoned flour and brown both sides in the heated oil, about 2 minutes per side. Remove from the pan and transfer to a 33 x 23cm (13 x 9in) baking dish. Set aside.

4. Add the remaining 1 tablespoon of oil and the sliced onion to the pan and cook for about 5 minutes, or until soft.

5. Meanwhile, in a small bowl, stir together 600ml (1 pint) of the chicken stock, the celery salt, the remaining ½ teaspoon salt, the pepper, and the remaining No. 1 All-Purpose Flour Blend.

6. Add the chicken stock mixture to the onion, and deglaze the pan, scraping off any tasty morsels with a wooden spoon. Add the cream of mushroom soup and the cream and stir well. If it is too thick, gradually add the remaining chicken stock until it's the consistency of gravy.

7. Pour the gravy on top of the meat, cover, transfer to the oven, and bake for 2 hours. Let cool slightly, and then serve.

Tip ....

This recipe was developed using condensed gluten-free mushroom soup. If you can only find thinner varieties of gluten-free mushroom soup, you may need to thicken the sauce at the end of cooking time. To do this, add No. 1 All-Purpose Flour Blend (see p24), 1 tbsp at a time, and return the sauce to a gentle simmer after each addition until it thickens to your liking. Taste to see if you also need more salt, then serve.

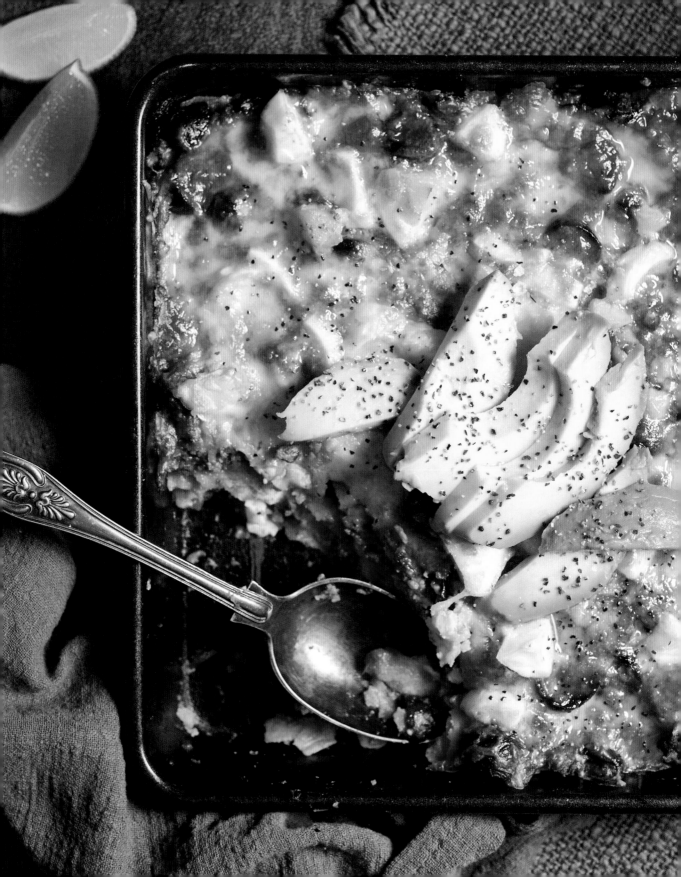

Serves:
6

Prep time:
20 minutes

Cook time:
35 minutes

1 tbsp avocado oil, or other vegetable oil, plus extra for greasing

1 small onion, chopped

2 garlic cloves, finely chopped or grated

450g (1lb) minced beef or turkey

285g can red enchilada sauce, available online, or in American and Mexican shops (gluten-free; see tip, below)

225g (8oz) tomato passata

½ tsp salt

130g can chopped or sliced black olives, drained

8–10 corn tortillas, quartered

3 hard-boiled large eggs, chopped

350g (12oz) Monterey Jack cheese, or mild Cheddar, grated

sour cream, guacamole or avocado slices, lime wedges, and hot sauce (optional), to serve

With all the flavours of enchiladas and the ease of a casserole, this recipe is great for busy nights during the week, and any that is left over gives you a delicious lunch the next day. My mum has been making this recipe for as long as I can remember.

Mama's Enchilada Pie

1. Preheat the oven to 180°C (160°C fan/350°F/Gas 4) and grease the base of a 20 or 23cm (8 or 9in) square baking dish.

2. In a large saucepan, heat the oil over a medium-high heat. Add the onion and sauté until soft, about 5 minutes. Add the garlic and cook for 30 seconds. Add the minced beef, breaking it up into small pieces, and cook until no longer pink in the middle. Drain off any fat.

3. Add the enchilada sauce, tomato passata, salt, and olives to the pan. Stir until combined and remove from the heat.

4. Place half the tortillas in the prepared baking dish, overlapping the pieces to cover the entire dish without any gaps. Pour half the meat mixture over the tortillas and spread evenly, followed by half the eggs and half the cheese.

5. Repeat the layers, ending with the remaining cheese. Bake, uncovered, for 30 minutes. Let rest for 5 minutes and then serve with the desired toppings.

Tip

Read the label! Most red enchilada sauces contain flour and aren't gluten-free. My favourite brand of gluten-free red enchilada sauce is Frontera, which is available online.

Serves:
4

Prep time:
15 minutes

Cook time:
15 minutes

Stir-fry typically contains soy sauce (which contains wheat), but this version uses tamari instead. The orange marmalade adds a touch of sweetness to balance out the ginger. Serve on top of rice and you'll be reminded of your favourite Chinese restaurant. My older son, a very picky eater, once said, "Mum, this is the best steak I've ever had!"

Chinese Takeaway Beef & Broccoli Stir-Fry

675g (1½lb) broccoli, cut into bite-sized florets

450g (1lb) flank steak (bavette), cut into 2.5cm x 5mm (1 x ¼in) slices

2 tbsp cornflour

1 garlic clove, finely chopped or grated

1 tsp grated fresh root ginger

½ tsp salt

dash of freshly ground black pepper

1 tbsp avocado oil, or other vegetable oil

1 tsp toasted sesame oil

4 tbsp marmalade

3 tbsp sweet chilli sauce

60ml (2fl oz) tamari, or coconut aminos

60ml (2fl oz) water

30g (1oz) roasted cashews

white rice, to serve

1. In a large saucepan, cover the broccoli florets with about 5cm (2in) of water. Cover and cook over a high heat for 5 minutes.

2. In a medium bowl, toss the steak with 1 tablespoon of the cornflour, the garlic, ginger, salt, and pepper until the steak is thoroughly coated.

3. In a large frying pan or wok, heat the avocado (or other vegetable oil) and sesame oils over a medium-high heat. Add the steak and stir-fry for 4–5 minutes or until almost cooked through. Reduce the heat to medium.

4. In a small bowl, whisk together the remaining 1 tablespoon of cornflour, the marmalade, sweet chilli sauce, tamari, and water. Whisk until well combined.

5. Add the broccoli and sauce to the frying pan or wok and mix well. Cover and simmer for 5 minutes, stirring frequently, until the sauce has slightly thickened. Stir in the cashews and serve over rice.

300g (10oz) gluten-free lasagne sheets (such as Doves Farm, or another brand of brown rice pasta), or 5–6 large courgettes, cut lengthways into 5mm (¼in) slices

1 tsp salt, plus extra if using courgettes

2 large eggs, lightly beaten

500g (1lb 2oz) full-fat cottage cheese

60g (2oz) freshly grated Parmesan cheese

1 tbsp dried parsley

½ tsp freshly ground black pepper

1kg (2¼lb) Mum's Famous Meat Sauce (see p82) or your favourite meaty pasta sauce

450g (1lb) mozzarella cheese, grated

I grew up eating this lasagne and now, with gluten-free lasagne sheets, or slices of courgette, I can still enjoy one of my childhood favourites. The home-made meat sauce, Mum's Famous Meat Sauce, is the secret here. It is absolutely worth the time and effort.

Meaty Lasagne

1. Preheat the oven to 190°C (170°C fan/375°F/Gas 5). If using pasta, cook the gluten-free lasagne sheets for 2 minutes less than directed by the the package instructions. Rinse immediately under cold water.

2. If using courgettes, sprinkle salt over the slices and place in a colander to drain for 15 minutes. Blot off any excess moisture with kitchen paper before using. Make sure the courgettes are as dry as possible.

3. In a medium bowl, beat the eggs. Add the cottage cheese, Parmesan, parsley, salt, and pepper. Stir until well combined.

4. Spread about 100g (3½oz) of the meat sauce in a 33 x 23cm (13 x 9in) baking dish. Layer half the lasagne sheets or courgette slices in the dish, overlapping them. Spread half the cottage cheese mixture over the lasagne or courgette, followed by one-third of the mozzarella cheese, and then top with half the remaining meat sauce. Repeat the layers using the remaining lasagne sheets or courgette slices, cottage cheese mixture, one-third of the mozzarella cheese, and remaining meat sauce. Finally, spread the remaining one-third of the mozzarella cheese on top.

5. Bake for 45 minutes, or until bubbly and the cheese is melted and golden brown. Let rest for 10–15 minutes before serving.

Store it

Store in an airtight container in the refrigerator for up to 5 days, or cut the lasagne into individual portions, place in airtight containers, and freeze for up to 3 months. Defrost in the refrigerator. Reheat in the microwave. You could also reheat frozen portions straight from the freezer, in an oven preheated to 180°C (160°C fan/ 350°F/Gas 4).

Makes:
about 24

Prep time:
10 minutes

Cook time:
25 minutes

A party would not be a party without my mum bringing her meatballs. They are definitely a crowd-pleaser and are great served over a big plate of gluten-free spaghetti, or as a canapé on a tray with toothpicks. They are also awesome served out of a slow-cooker, smothered in Mum's Famous Meat Sauce (see tip, below).

Home-Made Meatballs

1 tbsp avocado oil, or olive oil

1 small onion, chopped

3 garlic cloves, finely chopped or grated

450g (1lb) minced beef

450g (1lb) minced pork

50g (1¾oz) Home-Made Breadcrumbs (see p25) or store-bought plain gluten-free breadcrumbs

30g (1oz) freshly grated Parmesan cheese

2 tbsp tomato pasta sauce, or Mum's Famous Meat Sauce (see p82)

2 tsp dried parsley

1 tsp dried basil

½ tsp salt

¼ tsp freshly ground black pepper

1 large egg, lightly beaten

home-made tomato sauce, or shop-bought marinara sauce, to serve (optional)

1. Preheat the oven to 190°C (170°C fan/375°F/Gas 5). Line a baking tray with baking parchment. In a large sauté pan, heat the oil over a medium-high heat. Sauté the onion until soft and translucent, about 5 minutes. Add the garlic and cook for 1 minute more.

2. Transfer the cooked onion and garlic to a large bowl. Add the minced beef, minced pork, breadcrumbs, Parmesan, pasta sauce, parsley, basil, salt, pepper, and egg. Mix initially with a spoon, and then with your hands until combined; do not overmix or the meatballs will be tough.

3. Using a spoon, or your hands, roll the mixture into 5cm (2in) balls. Place the meatballs on the prepared baking tray and bake for 20–25 minutes. Remove from the oven and serve immediately, with tomato sauce, if you like.

Tip

To serve these with a sauce, once you've baked the meatballs, transfer them to a slow-cooker with Mum's Famous Meat Sauce (see p82) to cover, or 900g (2lb) shop-bought gluten-free marinara pasta sauce. Cook on low for 3 hours.

Store it

Lay the meatballs out on a baking tray and freeze. Once frozen, place them in a freezer bag or airtight container and freeze for up to 6 months. Defrost in the refrigerator, in the microwave, or place into a slow-cooker with sauce and reheat on low for 6 hours.

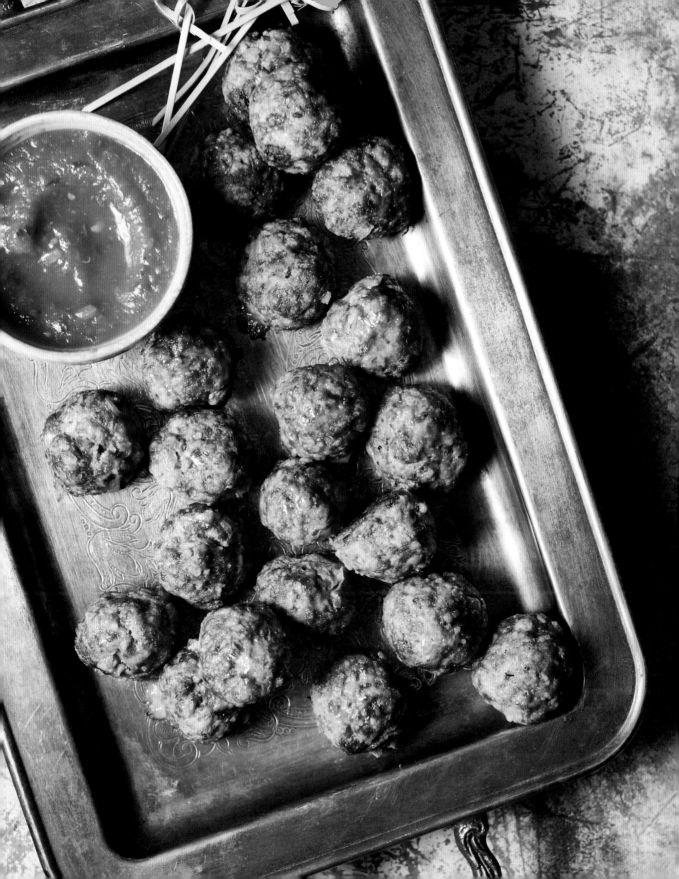

Makes:
about 2kg (4½lb),
or enough to serve
18 with pasta, or to make
1 quantity each Chicken
Parmesan and Meaty
Lasagne (see p54
and p79)

Prep time:
10 minutes

Cook time:
1½ hours (minimum)

2 tbsp avocado oil, or
    other vegetable oil
1 small onion, finely
    chopped
4 garlic cloves, finely
    chopped or grated
450g (1lb) minced beef or
    turkey
900g (2lb) tomato
    passata
170g can tomato purée
2 x 400g cans chopped
    tomatoes with herbs
1 tsp salt, or to taste
½ tsp freshly ground
    black pepper
1 tbsp dried basil
1 tbsp dried oregano
2 tbsp dried parsley
¼ tsp golden granulated
    sugar

My mum has been making this pasta sauce since I was a little girl and I have never found a ready-made sauce I liked as much. The longer the sauce simmers, the more flavoursome it will be. When I make a batch, I always use it over spaghetti and meatballs first, and then in Chicken Parmesan (see p54) or Meaty Lasagne (see p79).

Mum's Famous Meat Sauce

1. In a large heavy flameproof casserole dish or heavy-based saucepan, heat 1 tablespoon of the oil over a medium heat. Add the onion and sauté for about 5 minutes, or until soft and translucent. Add the garlic and sauté for 1 minute more.

2. Add the remaining 1 tablespoon of oil along with the minced beef or turkey, and cook, breaking it up into small pieces, until no longer pink.

3. Add the tomato passata and tomato purée. Stir well to combine.

4. Depending on whether or not you like chunks of tomatoes in your sauce, pulse the chopped tomatoes in a blender a few times to break up the large pieces, and then add to the casserole dish.

5. Add the salt, pepper, basil, oregano, parsley, and sugar to the pot. Stir well. Bring just to the boil, reduce the heat to low, cover, and simmer for a minimum of 1 hour, or even for the entire day. Salt to taste and serve.

Store it

Store in airtight containers in the refrigerator for up to 5 days. This sauce freezes well. I like to freeze it in multiple 225g (8oz) containers; that way I always have some sauce ready and it can be used as an individual portion, or I can defrost a couple of containers for the whole family.

Serves:
6

Prep time:
20 minutes

Cook time:
1 hour 20 minutes

Special equipment:
probe thermometer

This recipe is for my dad and father-in-law: meatloaf is their favourite meal! Add a couple of side dishes of mashed potatoes and gravy and they'd both be in heaven. This meatloaf is loaded with flavour and uses gluten-free crackers. It's crispy on the outside and moist on the inside without being mushy.

Meatloaf
with Balsamic Glaze

50g (1¾oz) gluten-free crackers

1 tbsp avocado oil, or other vegetable oil

50g (1¾oz) finely chopped onion

4 garlic cloves, finely chopped or grated

2 large eggs, lightly beaten

900g (2lb) minced beef

60g (2oz) freshly grated Parmesan cheese

1 tsp dried parsley

3 tbsp tomato ketchup

2 tbsp Worcestershire sauce (gluten-free)

½ tbsp Dijon mustard

1½ tsp salt

½ tsp freshly ground black pepper

½ tsp paprika

For the glaze

115g (4oz) tomato ketchup

1 tbsp balsamic vinegar

3 tbsp light brown sugar

½ tsp garlic powder

¼ tsp onion powder

¼ tsp freshly ground black pepper

¼ tsp salt

1. Preheat the oven to 200°C (180°C fan/400°F/Gas 6). Place the crackers in a resealable bag and use a rolling pin to crush them into fine crumbs.

2. Make the glaze. In a small bowl, stir together all the ingredients and set aside until needed.

3. In a small pan, heat the oil over a medium heat and sauté the onion until soft and translucent. Add the garlic and cook for 1 minute more. Set aside and let cool.

4. Put the eggs in a large bowl. Add the onion, minced beef, Parmesan, parsley, ketchup, Worcestershire sauce, mustard, salt, pepper, paprika, and cracker crumbs. Mix with your hands until just combined; do not overmix.

5. Transfer the meat mixture to a 23 x 12.5cm (9 x 5in) loaf tin and lightly press down. Brush half the glaze evenly over the top of the loaf, reserving the other half for later.

6. Bake the meatloaf for 40 minutes. Remove the tin from the oven and spread half the remaining glaze evenly over the top. Bake for an additional 20–30 minutes or until the internal temperature reaches at least 71°C (160°F). Pour off any grease that has accumulated and reserve. Let rest for 10 minutes.

7. While the meatloaf is resting, make a sauce to serve. In a small pan, mix 2 tablespoons of the poured-off juices from the tin with the remaining glaze. Simmer until heated through. Remove the loaf from the pan, slice, and serve with the sauce.

Tip ....

If you love the crispier outer edges of the meatloaf like I do, then prepare this recipe as mini loaves or in a cupcake tin. Bake the smaller loaves for 25 minutes, brush with half the remaining glaze, and bake for 10 minutes more, or until the internal temperature reaches 71°C (160°F).

Flour-Free Sides & Soups

....

Serves:
4

Prep time:
10 minutes

Cook time:
20 minutes

Going gluten-free is easier when you eat lots of veggies to fill up, but I get tired of plain, steamed broccoli over and over again. This roasted recipe has so much more flavour and makes a nice change from the usual. My favourite part is the crispy Parmesan. It's prepared in one bowl and the baking tray is lined, so it's easy to make and clean up.

Roasted Tenderstem Broccoli

3 bunches of Tenderstem broccoli, about 675g (1½lb) in total

3 tbsp avocado oil, or olive oil

1 tbsp lemon juice

3 garlic cloves, finely chopped or grated

½ tsp salt

¼ tsp freshly ground black pepper

85g (3oz) freshly grated Parmesan cheese

1. Preheat the oven to 220°C (200°C fan/425°F/Gas 7) and line a baking tray with baking parchment. Wash and trim the broccoli and pat dry with kitchen paper.

2. In a large bowl, toss the broccoli with the oil until all the pieces are coated. Add the lemon juice and toss until well distributed.

3. Add the garlic, salt, pepper, and 60g (2oz) of the Parmesan. Toss until well combined.

4. Evenly spread the broccoli on the prepared baking tray. Sprinkle the remaining Parmesan on top.

5. Bake for 20 minutes, or until the desired doneness. Serve immediately.

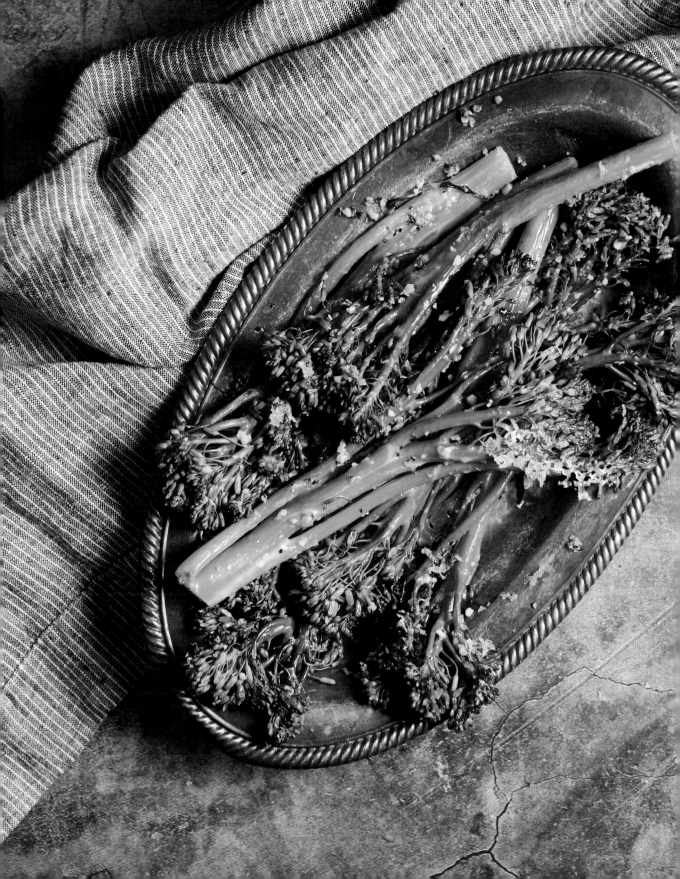

Serves:
4

Prep time:
10 minutes

Cook time:
35 minutes

I grew up eating Brussels sprouts with canned cheese sauce poured on top: so good! When I tried to introduce Brussels sprouts to my family, they looked at me like I had lost it. No interest! Determined to cook a recipe my family would tolerate, I developed this salty, sweet, crispy dish. Not only do they tolerate it, but they actually really like it.

Maple Bacon Brussels Sprouts

450g (1lb) Brussels sprouts
1½ tbsp avocado oil, or other vegetable oil
½ tsp salt
freshly ground black pepper
4 bacon rashers
1 tbsp pure maple syrup

1. Preheat the oven to 220°C (200°C fan/425°F/Gas 7). Wash the Brussels sprouts and drain. Trim the ends, and cut each sprout in half.

2. In a large bowl, toss the Brussels sprout halves with the oil, salt, and pepper. Spread them out on a baking tray lined with baking parchment.

3. Roast the Brussels sprouts for 20–25 minutes or until crispy and golden brown, stirring once halfway through the cooking time.

4. While the Brussels sprouts are roasting, in a large sauté pan, cook the bacon over a medium heat until crispy. Remove the bacon, and reserve 2 tablespoons of its rendered fat in the pan, draining the rest. Chop the bacon.

5. Once the Brussels sprouts are ready, heat the reserved 2 tablespoons bacon fat in the same sauté pan. Add the Brussels sprouts and toss to coat evenly. Add the chopped bacon and cook until heated through, 3–5 minutes.

6. Add the maple syrup and toss to coat. Cook for an additional 1–2 minutes. Serve immediately.

Tip ....
You can roast and cook the Brussels sprouts and bacon up to 1 day in advance and store in the refrigerator. When ready to serve, follow steps 5 and 6.

Serves:
about 10

Prep time:
30 minutes, plus
2 hours to chill

Cook time:
10 minutes

As a child standing at a restaurant salad bar, I always chose macaroni salad as a side dish. After going gluten-free, a trip to Hawaii – where macaroni salad appeared at every turn – motivated me to create my own recipe. I spent a full week making Hawaiian macaroni salad until I perfected it, and perfection this salad is.

Hawaiian Macaroni Salad

450g (1lb) gluten-free brown rice macaroni

60ml (2fl oz) apple cider vinegar

550ml (1 pint) whole milk

520g (1lb 3oz) mayonnaise

2½ tbsp light brown sugar

1½ tbsp pickle juice (from a jar of gluten-free pickles/gherkins)

½ tsp freshly ground black pepper

15g (½oz) grated onion

30g (1oz) grated carrot

75g (2¾oz) finely chopped celery

salt

1. Bring a large pot of salted water to the boil and cook the pasta for 2–5 minutes less than directed by the package instructions; it needs to be al dente as it will absorb the sauce later. Drain and rinse under hot water immediately.

2. Pour the pasta back into the pot and add the vinegar. Stir until it's evenly distributed and absorbed. Cool for 10 minutes.

3. While the pasta is cooling, in a small bowl, whisk together 360ml (12fl oz) of the milk, 225g (8oz) of the mayonnaise, the brown sugar, pickle juice, and pepper.

4. Add the milk and mayonnaise mixture to the pasta and stir until combined. Cool completely in the refrigerator, about 1 hour, stirring from time to time.

5. Add the onion, carrot, celery, remaining milk, and remaining mayonnaise to the pasta. Mix until evenly distributed. Cover and refrigerate for at least 1 hour, stirring from time to time. It will be a little runny at first, but as the pasta absorbs the sauce, it will thicken up. Taste and add more salt if desired. Serve chilled.

Store it
Store in an airtight container in the refrigerator for up to 5 days.

Tips
For day-to-day use, I normally use an avocado oil-based mayonnaise. However, for this recipe, I have found that Hellmann's tastes best.

This recipe is great to make a day in advance, because it tastes better the longer it sits.

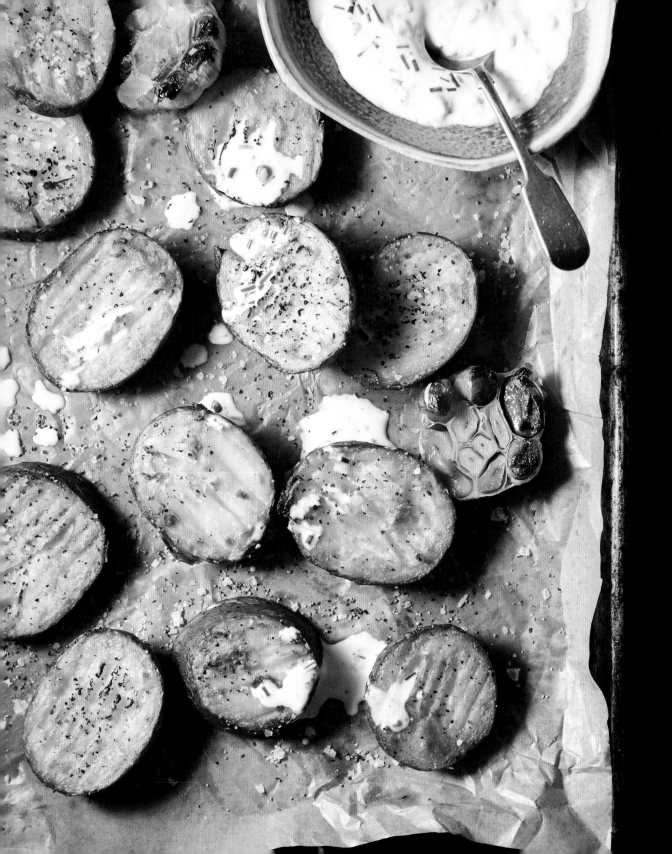

The combination of sweetness from the potatoes with salty tartness from the aioli is a match made in heaven. I prefer to roast the garlic here, but raw garlic works just as well. White-fleshed sweet potatoes, if you can find them, are only slightly sweet, so if you normally don't go for sweet potatoes, give this dish a try: it might change your mind.

Smashed Sweet Potatoes
with Easy Garlic Aioli

3 large sweet potatoes, ideally white-fleshed, about 900g (2lb) in total

1 tsp salt, plus extra for seasoning

olive oil, for brushing

freshly ground black pepper

For the aioli

85g (3oz) mayonnaise

1 tbsp olive oil

1½ tsp lemon juice

1 tbsp chopped chives

¼ tsp salt

½–1 tsp chopped capers

2 garlic cloves, finely chopped or grated, or roasted and smashed (see note, below)

1. Slice the unpeeled potatoes into 1.25cm (½in) rounds.

2. Bring a large saucepan of water to the boil over a high heat. Add the measured salt and the sliced potatoes, then reduce the heat to a simmer. Gently cook for 20–25 minutes or until very soft. Drain the potatoes and let cool.

3. Preheat the oven to 220°C (200°C fan/425°F/Gas 7) and arrange the cooled potato slices on a baking tray lined with baking parchment. Using a fork, gently smash the potatoes, keeping the skins intact as much as possible.

4. Brush olive oil onto each potato slice, and then sprinkle salt and pepper over. Bake for 15 minutes.

5. Gently flip each potato slice. Brush with more olive oil and sprinkle with more salt and pepper. Bake for an additional 15 minutes. If you'd like them extra crispy, place the baking tray on the top oven shelf and grill for 1–2 minutes, watching the potatoes closely to prevent burning. Serve the potato slices immediately with the aioli.

Easy Garlic Aioli: In a small bowl, whisk together the mayonnaise, olive oil, lemon juice, chives, salt, capers, garlic, and a dash of pepper. Whisk until well combined. Refrigerate until ready to serve.

Roasted Garlic: Preheat the oven to 200°C (180°C fan/400°F/Gas 6). Peel off any loose skin that is hanging from the entire bulb, but be sure to leave the skins on the cloves. Keeping the entire bulb intact, cut 5mm–1.25cm (¼–½in) off the top, exposing the inside of each clove. Place the bulb on a piece of foil. Drizzle a small amount of olive oil over the entire bulb. Enclose the bulb with the foil and bake for 30–40 minutes or until the cloves are extremely soft and spreadable. This recipe only calls for 2 cloves of garlic; reserve the extra roasted garlic cloves for another use, such as spreading on warmed bread.

Serves:
8

Prep time:
20 minutes

Cook time:
50 minutes

1 tsp salt

1 small onion, chopped

1.6kg (3½lb) Maris Piper potatoes, peeled and cut into 1.25cm (½in) cubes

70g (1½oz) salted butter

1 garlic clove, very finely chopped or grated

4 tbsp No. 1 All-Purpose Flour Blend (see p24)

480ml (16fl oz) whole milk

dash of freshly ground black pepper

350g (12oz) strong Cheddar cheese, grated

My mum has been making this recipe for as long as I can remember, and it is not Christmas or Easter without this side dish on the table. It's my absolute favourite way to eat potatoes. They are exceptional alongside ham, for dipping in the cheesy sauce.

Mum's Cheesy Potatoes

1. Preheat the oven to 190°C (170°C fan/375°F/Gas 5). Bring a large saucepan of water to the boil. Add ½ teaspoon salt, the chopped onion, and the potatoes. Cook for 10 minutes. Drain and rinse under cold water.

2. In a large saucepan, melt the butter over a medium heat. Sauté the garlic until fragrant, about 30 seconds. Add the flour and stir for 30 seconds. Add the milk and cook, stirring constantly, until the sauce boils.

3. Add the remaining ½ teaspoon salt, pepper, and the Cheddar. Stir until the cheese is melted. Add the potatoes and stir to combine.

4. Pour into a 2.5 litre (4½ pint) ovenproof dish and bake, uncovered, for 30 minutes, or until bubbly and the potatoes are tender when poked with a fork. Let sit for 5–10 minutes before serving.

Tips ....

These potatoes are not only amazing served with ham, but also Brussels sprouts, asparagus, or broccoli. The vegetables taste great dipped in the cheese sauce.

Serves:
10

Prep time:
10 minutes

Cook time:
45 minutes

370g (13oz) long-grain
   white rice
450ml (15fl oz) sour cream
200g can chopped mild
   green chillies
vegetable oil, for greasing
115–225g (4–8oz) Cheddar
   cheese, grated, to taste
225g (8oz) Monterey Jack
   cheese, or mild Cheddar,
   grated

This is another recipe from my mother-in-law that is served at almost every holiday dinner or family barbecue. It is naturally all gluten-free, but it is loved by so many that I just had to include it in this book. I love eating any leftovers for lunch the next day.

Cheesy Rice Casserole

1. Preheat the oven to 180°C (160°C fan/350°F/Gas 4). Cook the rice according to the package instructions.

2. In a small bowl, stir together the sour cream and chopped chillies.

3. Grease a 2.5 litre (4½ pint) ovenproof dish. Evenly spread out a layer of half the rice and lightly press down. Spread half the sour cream mixture on top. Sprinkle half of both cheeses on top of the sour cream. Repeat the layers once more, using the remaining rice, sour cream mixture, and then cheese.

4. Bake for 30–35 minutes or until the cheese is melted and bubbly. Serve immediately.

Serves:
4–6

Prep time:
20 minutes

Cook time:
20 minutes

A's Burgers, a fast-food restaurant in my California town, has the best fried courgettes, especially when dipped in their ranch dressing. Growing up we would go to A's Burgers about once a week just for this. My recipe is not only gluten-free, but also baked instead of fried so you can enjoy your "fried" courgettes without the guilt.

Oven "Fried" Courgettes

80g (2¾oz) No. 1 All-Purpose Flour Blend (see p24)

3 large eggs

200g (7oz) Home-Made Breadcrumbs (see p25) or store-bought plain gluten-free breadcrumbs

60g (2oz) freshly grated Parmesan cheese

2 tsp dried parsley

2 tsp salt

½ tsp freshly ground black pepper

1 tsp garlic powder

3 medium courgettes, cut into 5mm (¼in) thick rounds

avocado oil, or light cooking spray, to coat

Home-made ranch dressing (see p52, step 4) or another shop-bought dipping sauce, to serve

chopped chives, to serve

1. Preheat the oven to 200°C (180°C fan/400°F/Gas 6). Line 2 baking trays with baking parchment.

2. Prepare 3 shallow dishes. In the first, place the No. 1 All-Purpose Flour Blend. In the second, lightly beat the eggs. In the third, stir together the breadcrumbs, Parmesan, parsley, salt, pepper, and garlic powder.

3. Coat the courgette slices in the flour, then in the eggs, and finally roll them around and press into the breadcrumbs to coat completely. Place each coated courgette round on the prepared baking trays. Once they're all prepared, spray the tops of the slices with oil or cooking spray to help them crisp up.

4. Bake for 10 minutes. Flip and spray the other sides of each slice with oil or cooking spray. Bake for an additional 10 minutes, or until the courgette slices are soft and the breadcrumbs are golden brown and crispy. Serve immediately with ranch dressing sprinkled with chives, for dipping.

Air Fryer Method: Make these extra-crispy in half the time using an air fryer. Prepare steps 1 to 4 as written. However, spray both sides of the courgette slices before cooking. In the fryer basket, arrange the courgette slices in an even layer (do not overlap), working in batches as needed. Cook them at 200°C (400°F) for 9 minutes, and serve immediately.

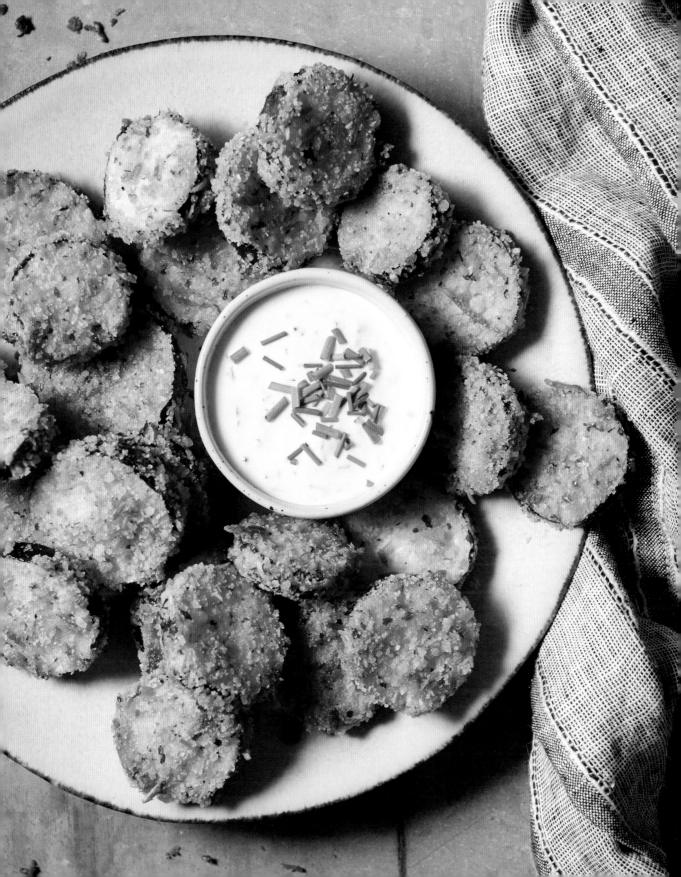

Serves:
16

Prep time:
10 minutes

Cook time:
6 hours

It wouldn't be a family barbecue without Phil's beans. Phil, a long-time neighbour of my in-laws, was a fireman and would take whatever ingredients were available at his fire station and make a pot of beans. From his creations came this recipe. It's not chilli and it's not baked beans: it's "Phil's Beans", in a category of its own. They are amazing!

Phil's Fire Station Beans

350g (12oz) sausagemeat

2 x 400g cans gluten-free baked beans, undrained

2 x 400g cans kidney beans, drained

400g can cannellini beans, undrained

400g can chilli beans in chilli sauce (ideally green chilli sauce, such as Ranch Style Beans with Jalapeño Peppers, available online), undrained

1 onion, chopped

225g (8oz) white or brown mushrooms, sliced

3 celery sticks, chopped

40g (1¼oz) light brown sugar

75g (2¾oz) tomato ketchup

2 tbsp American yellow mustard

1. In a large frying pan, brown the sausagemeat, breaking it up into small pieces. Drain off the fat. Put the sausage in a slow-cooker.

2. Add all the remaining ingredients to the slow-cooker and stir to distribute evenly. Cover and cook on low for 4–6 hours. Serve immediately.

Store it

Store in an airtight container in the refrigerator for up to 5 days, or in the freezer for up to 3 months. Reheat on the hob.

Tips

If you want to speed up the cooking time after browning the sausagemeat, add all the ingredients to a very large saucepan and simmer over a low heat for 2–3 hours.

Serves:
at least 20 people
as a starter

Prep time:
15 minutes

Cook time:
4 hours (minimum)

You knew what day it was when you walked into the house and smelled this soup: my husband's grandma Helen was famous for her split pea soup on Christmas Eve. She would start cooking it when she woke up, and it would simmer all day. She always served it as a starter while the finishing touches were being put to the dinner.

Grandma Helen's Split Pea Soup

400g (14oz) dried green split peas

480ml (16fl oz) chicken stock

2.4 litres (4 pints) filtered water

1 smoked ham hock

1 onion, chopped

½ tsp garlic powder

½ tsp dried oregano

½ tsp freshly ground black pepper

1 bay leaf

190g (6½oz) carrots, finely sliced

100g (3½oz) celery, chopped

1. In a large saucepan, combine the peas, chicken stock, water, ham hock, onion, garlic powder, oregano, pepper, and bay leaf.

2. Cook, uncovered, for 1½ hours at a rolling boil, stirring occasionally.

3. Remove the ham hock, trim off and discard the skin, fat, and gristle, and chop the meat. Return the ham pieces to the pot.

4. Stir in the carrots and celery. Simmer over a low heat, covered, for 2½ hours, or even for the remainder of the day. Serve hot.

Store it

Store in an airtight container in the refrigerator for up to 5 days, or freeze individual portions in airtight containers for up to 3 months. Reheat on the hob over a low heat, or in the microwave.

Tips

The longer this soup simmers, the more it will thicken. If you like your split pea soup on the thicker side, then simmer it for as long as possible.

If you like your soup extra-meaty, chop 1–2 gammon steaks and add them with the carrots and celery.

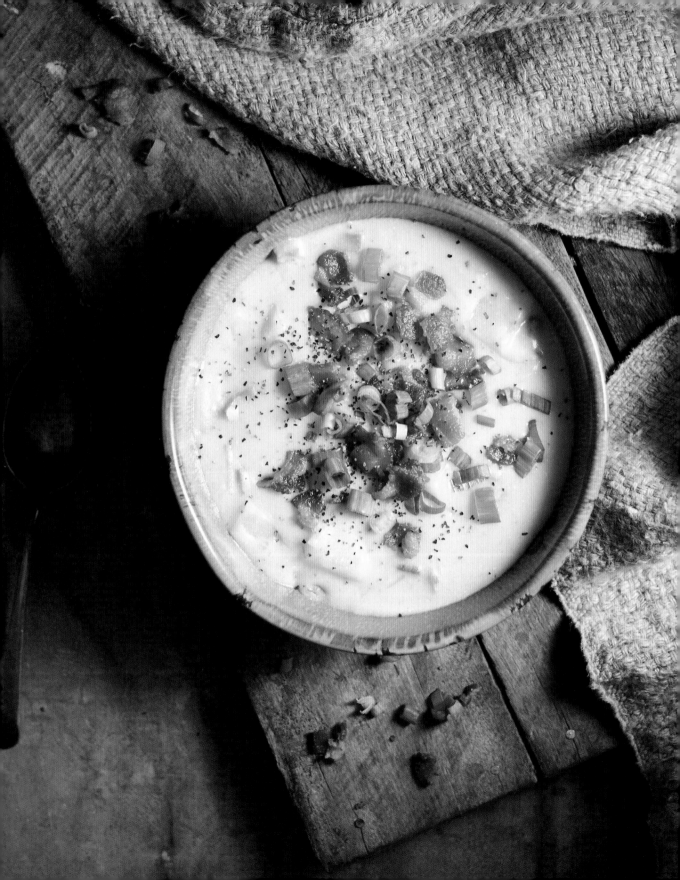

Serves:
8

Prep time:
15 minutes

Cook time:
35 minutes

A loaded baked potato with sour cream, bacon, chives, and Cheddar cheese is one of my favourite things to eat for dinner. This soup recipe combines all of those flavours into one giant pot. It is – truly – the ultimate comfort food.

Loaded Baked Potato Soup

350g (12oz) bacon, chopped into lardons

100g (3½oz) chopped onion

115g (4oz) salted butter

80g (2¾oz) No. 1 All-Purpose Flour Blend (see p24)

900ml (1½ pints) chicken stock

900ml (1½ pints) whole milk

900g (2lb) Maris Piper potatoes, peeled and cubed

4 spring onions, finely sliced

140g (5oz) ham, chopped

350g (12oz) strong Cheddar cheese, grated

240ml (8fl oz) sour cream

1 tsp salt

½ tsp freshly ground black pepper

1. Heat a large saucepan or heavy flameproof casserole dish over a medium-high heat. Add the bacon lardons and cook until crispy. Remove the bacon and drain off all but 1 tablespoon of the fat.

2. Cook the onion in the bacon fat for about 5 minutes, or until translucent.

3. Add the butter and melt. Whisk in the No. 1 All-Purpose Flour Blend and cook, whisking constantly, for 1 minute.

4. Gradually whisk in the chicken stock and milk. Cook, whisking constantly, until slightly thickened, 1–2 minutes. Stir in the potatoes, half the spring onions, and the chopped ham.

5. Bring to the boil, reduce the heat, and simmer, covered, for 15–20 minutes or until the potatoes are tender when pierced with a fork.

6. Stir in 250g (9oz) of the Cheddar, the sour cream, and half the bacon. Season with the salt and pepper. Serve immediately, topped with the remaining spring onions, bacon, and Cheddar.

Serves:
8

Prep time:
15 minutes

Cook time:
1 hour 10 minutes

Have you ever craved Mexican food but wanted the comfort of a bowl of soup? Then this recipe is exactly what you're looking for. It was introduced to me by my mother-in-law, and I made a few changes to make it gluten-free. This one-pot meal is easy to make, and everyone can customize their own bowl with an array of toppings.

Taco Soup

1 tbsp avocado oil, or olive oil

50g (1¾oz) chopped onion

900g (2lb) minced beef or turkey

400g can chopped tomatoes with chilli

2 x 400g cans pinto beans, undrained

400g can black beans, undrained

400g can kidney beans, drained

400g can sweetcorn, drained

400g can chopped tomatoes

400g can chopped tomatoes with green chillies, undrained (available online), or 1 extra can chopped tomatoes with chilli

130g can chopped green chillies

115g can sliced black olives, drained

2 tbsp Home-Made Taco Seasoning (see right) or shop-bought gluten-free taco seasoning

25g (1oz) ranch seasoning mix (gluten-free; such as Hidden Valley, available online)

grated Monterey Jack or mild Cheddar cheese, sour cream, jalapeños, coriander, and tortilla chips (optional), to serve

1. In a large saucepan or heavy flameproof casserole dish, heat the oil over a medium heat. Add the onion and minced meat and cook until the meat is no longer pink, breaking it up into small pieces.

2. While the meat is cooking, put the chopped tomatoes with chilli with their juices in a food processor or blender. Pulse a few times to break up the large pieces of tomato.

3. Stir the processed tomatoes into the pot with the pinto beans, black beans, kidney beans, sweetcorn, chopped tomatoes, chopped tomatoes with green chillies, green chillies, black olives, taco seasoning, and ranch seasoning mix. Simmer, covered, over a low heat for 1 hour. Serve immediately with the desired toppings.

Slow-Cooker Method: First cook the onion and meat in a sauté pan, then add to a slow-cooker. Stir in the remaining ingredients. Cook on low for 5–6 hours, or on high for 2–3 hours.

Store it
Store in airtight containers in the refrigerator for up to 5 days, or freeze individual portions in airtight containers for up to 3 months. Reheat on the hob or in the microwave.

Home-Made Taco Seasoning:

4 tsp ground cumin

4 tsp paprika

2 tsp dried ground onion

2 tsp garlic salt

1 tsp dried granulated garlic

1 tsp chilli powder

½ tsp cayenne, or to taste

4 tsp dried oregano

1 tsp freshly ground black pepper

2 tsp golden granulated sugar (optional)

In a small bowl, mix together all the ingredients. This recipe makes about 180g (6oz). I always have it on hand for whenever we make tacos, because many packaged seasonings have added preservatives, or are not gluten-free.

Serves:
8–10

Prep time:
10 minutes

Cook time:
1 hour

2 tbsp avocado oil, or olive oil

675–900g (1½–2lb) pork loin, cut into 2.5cm (1in) pieces

1 tbsp No. 1 All-Purpose Flour Blend (see p24)

½ onion, chopped

3 garlic cloves, finely chopped or grated

120ml (4fl oz) dry white wine (or chicken stock)

1.5 litres (2¾ pints) chicken stock

1 bay leaf

2 tsp salt

½ tsp freshly ground black pepper

2 x 115g cans chopped green chillies, undrained

125g (4½oz) sliced carrots

675g (1½lb) Maris Piper potatoes, white-fleshed sweet potatoes, or turnips, peeled and cut into 2.5cm (1in) pieces

400g can pinto beans, drained

400g can cannellini beans, drained

1 tsp dried thyme

½ tsp ground cumin

½ tsp ground coriander

1 tsp dried oregano

bunch of kale (optional), coarse ribs stripped out, leaves chopped

grated mild cheese, sour cream, coriander, chopped avocado, and chopped jalapeños (optional), to serve

This twist on a home-made stew has a bit of a Mexican flair to it. The cumin and chopped green chillies provide the perfect blend of flavours. Like chilli, it is fun to set up a topping bar when serving this soup. It tastes great with sour cream, grated mild cheese, coriander, jalapeños, or sliced avocados on top.

Mexican Pork Stew

1. In a large saucepan or heavy flameproof casserole, heat 1 tablespoon of the oil over a medium-high heat. In a large bowl, season the pork with salt and pepper, and toss to combine. Add the No. 1 All-Purpose Flour Blend and toss to thoroughly coat. Brown the pork in the hot oil.

2. Remove the pork from the pot. Add the remaining 1 tablespoon oil and sauté the onion for about 5 minutes, or until translucent. Add the garlic and cook for 1 minute more.

3. Add the wine and deglaze the pan by scraping with a wooden spoon. Add the stock, bay leaf, salt, pepper, green chillies, carrots, potatoes, pinto beans, cannellini beans, thyme, cumin, coriander, and oregano, along with the pork.

4. Bring the soup to the boil, reduce the heat and simmer, covered, for 40 minutes.

5. If using, add the kale and simmer for an additional 10 minutes. Serve immediately with the desired toppings.

Store it ···

Store in an airtight container in the refrigerator for up to 5 days, or freeze individual portions in airtight containers for up to 3 months. Reheat on the hob, or in the microwave.

Perfect Pizzas & Breads

Makes:
1 x 28cm (11in) crust
or 2 x 20cm (8in) crusts

Prep time:
35 minutes

Cook time:
15 minutes

Special equipment:
cooking thermometer

200g (7oz) brown rice
    flour
1¼ tsp fast-action dried
    yeast (or active dry
    yeast; see tip, below)
1½ tsp salt
1 tsp Italian seasoning
2 tsp xanthan gum
½ tsp garlic powder
¼ tsp onion powder
2 tsp golden granulated
    sugar
180ml (6fl oz) warm
    water at 40–43°C
    (105–110°F)
1 tbsp olive oil, plus extra
    for brushing
2 tsp apple cider vinegar
90g (3¼oz) tapioca flour

Frozen pizzas, or those delivered to your home, just aren't the same when gluten-free, and home-made options typically involve hours of labour. So, like most other foods I miss, I created my own. This pizza crust is actually really easy to make and does not take long at all. It has also been approved by both my kids!

Easy Peasy Pizza Crust

1. Preheat the oven to 220°C (200°C fan/425°F/Gas 7) with a pizza stone or heavy baking tray inside the oven. (If you prefer to use active dry yeast, you will need to proof the yeast now; see tip, below.) In a stand mixer fitted with the paddle attachment, or in a large bowl, whisk together 80g (2¾oz) of the brown rice flour, the fast-action dried yeast (if using), salt, Italian seasoning, xanthan gum, garlic powder, onion powder, and sugar until well combined.

2. Turn the mixer to its slowest speed and add the warm water, olive oil, and vinegar. Slowly add the remaining brown rice flour and the tapioca flour. Mix on low speed for 1–2 minutes, or until the dough comes together and pulls away from the sides of the bowl. Let rest for 10 minutes.

3. Rub a little bit of oil on your hands to prevent the dough from sticking. Form the dough into a disc (or 2 discs if making 2 pizzas) and place between 2 sheets of baking parchment. Roll the dough out into a 3–5mm (⅛–¼in) thick circle, about 28cm (11in) in diameter, or 2 discs of the same thickness measuring 20cm (8in) in diameter. Remove the top sheet of parchment. Using a fork, gently poke holes around the whole crust. Brush the entire crust with olive oil. Cover it with the top sheet of baking parchment and let rest for 10 minutes.

4. Remove the top sheet of parchment. Using the bottom sheet, transfer the crust onto the stone or baking tray, keeping the parchment under the crust.

5. Par-bake for 15 minutes. Remove the crust and immediately brush the edges with water. The crust is now ready for your favourite toppings.

6. Once you've added the toppings, brush the edges with olive oil and bake for 12–15 minutes or until the cheese is golden brown.

Store it

After you've par-baked and cooled the crust, store in an airtight container in the freezer for up to 3 months. When ready to use, put your toppings directly on the frozen pizza and then bake. No need to defrost first.

Tip

To proof active dry yeast, stir the yeast into 120ml (4fl oz) of the warm water, along with 1 teaspoon of the sugar. (Add the remaining sugar with the dry mixture and the remaining water with the wet ingredients.) Let sit for 5 minutes, or until foamy. Add the yeast mixture along with the rest of the wet ingredients.

Makes:
1 x 28cm (11in) pizza

Prep time:
10 minutes

Cook time:
15 minutes

1 par-baked Easy Peasy
    Pizza Crust (see left)
bottle of shop-bought
    barbecue sauce
    (gluten-free)
225g (8oz) grated
    mozzarella cheese
75g (2½oz) cooked
    chicken, cubed
1 tbsp chopped red onion
1 tbsp chopped coriander
olive oil, for brushing

Once I eventually caved and tried a barbecue pizza, I was hooked. As soon as I developed my gluten-free pizza crust, barbecue chicken was the first pizza I created. The barbecue sauce, onion, and coriander deliver a great combination of flavours. If you're looking to mix up pizza night, this is a great recipe to try.

Barbecue Chicken Pizza

1. Preheat the oven to 200°C (180°C fan/400°F/Gas 6) with a pizza stone or heavy baking tray inside the oven. Place the par-baked pizza crust on a piece of baking parchment for easy transfer. Spread the barbecue sauce all over the crust, leaving a bit uncovered around the perimeter.

2. Top with three-quarters of the mozzarella, all the chicken, onion, and coriander. Sprinkle the remaining mozzarella on top.

3. Brush olive oil around the outside edge of the crust. Place the pizza directly on the preheated pizza stone or baking tray. Bake for 12–15 minutes or until the crust is golden brown and the cheese has melted. Slice and serve hot.

Tip ....
Serve with a side of ranch dressing for dipping (see p52, step 4 for my home-made version). This pizza would also taste great with shredded pork instead of chicken.

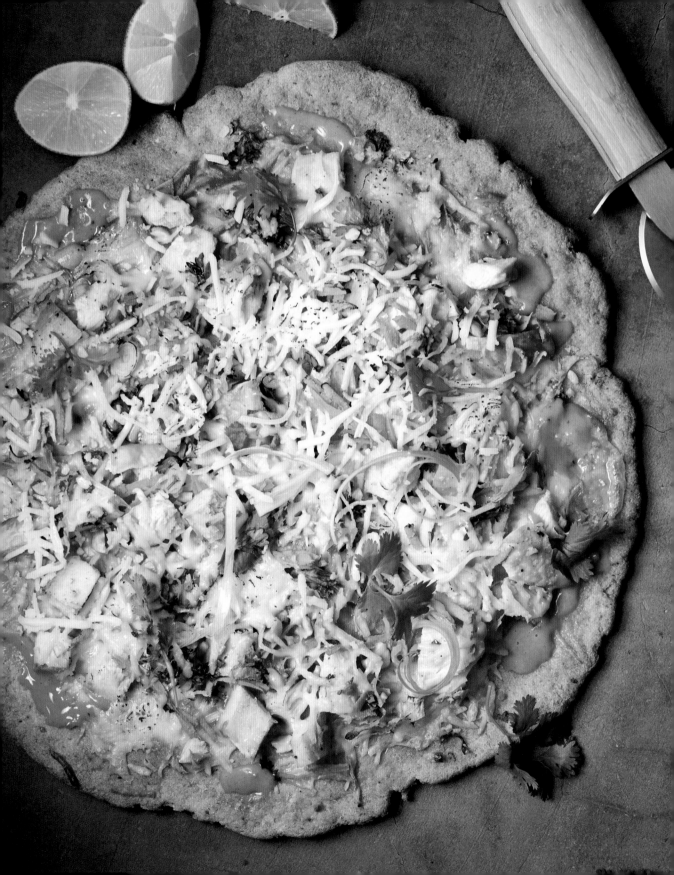

Makes:
1 x 28cm (11in) pizza

Prep time:
10 minutes

Cook time:
15 minutes

1 par-baked Easy Peasy
    Pizza Crust (see p104)
175–225g (6–8oz) grated
    mozzarella cheese,
    to taste
100g (3½oz) cooked
    chicken, cubed
1 small carrot, grated
1 spring onion, chopped
1 tbsp chopped coriander
1 tbsp chopped peanuts
olive oil, for brushing
lime wedges, to serve
    (optional)

For the peanut sauce

60g (2oz) smooth peanut
    butter (unsweetened)
1 tbsp tamari, or coconut
    aminos
⅛ tsp ground ginger
¼ tsp garlic powder
½ tbsp rice wine vinegar
1 tbsp light brown sugar
1 tsp sweet chilli sauce
    (gluten-free)
1 tsp lime juice
3 tbsp water, plus extra
    if needed

A famous California-based commercial pizza company makes a Thai chicken pizza, and it was my favourite when I was still eating gluten. Here is my version of that pizza. The creamy gluten-free peanut sauce is quick and easy to make. The many different flavours and textures in this pizza all combine to create one delicious meal!

Thai Chicken Pizza

1. Preheat the oven to 200°C (180°C fan/400°F/Gas 6) with a pizza stone or heavy baking tray inside the oven. Place the par-baked pizza crust on a piece of baking parchment for easy transfer. Prepare the peanut sauce. In a small bowl, whisk together all the ingredients. If the sauce is too thick, slowly whisk in more water 1 teaspoon at a time until you reach the desired consistency.

2. Spread the peanut sauce all over the par-baked pizza crust, leaving a bit uncovered around the perimeter. Top with three-quarters of the mozzarella (to taste), the chicken, carrot, spring onion, coriander, and peanuts. Sprinkle the remaining mozzarella on top.

3. Brush olive oil around the outside edge of the crust. Place the pizza directly on the preheated pizza stone or baking tray. Bake for 12–15 minutes or until the crust is golden brown and the cheese has melted. Slice and serve hot, with lime wedges, if you like.

Tip ....
Dip the pizza in any leftover peanut sauce, a sweet chilli sauce, or your favourite hot sauce.

Makes:
1 x 28cm (11in) pizza

Prep time:
10 minutes

Cook time:
15 minutes

1 par-baked Easy Peasy
Pizza Crust (see p104)

175g (6oz) refried beans

50–75g (1¾–2½oz)
Monterey Jack cheese,
or mild Cheddar, grated

50–75g (1¾–2½oz)
Cheddar cheese, grated

100g (3½oz) cooked
chicken, cubed

2 tbsp chopped black
olives

1–2 tbsp chopped
coriander

1 plum tomato, finely
chopped

1 spring onion, chopped

olive oil, for brushing

sour cream, tomato salsa,
pickled jalapeños, or
guacamole (optional),
to serve

This pizza is so versatile because you can use so many different ingredients, many of which I usually have on hand in my pantry. My kids like it with just beans and cheese, while my husband and I pack on the ingredients as if the pizza was a plate of loaded nachos. A build-your-own Mexican pizza is a fun meal to create with a group.

Mexican Pizza

1. Preheat the oven to 200°C (180°C fan/400°F/Gas 6) with a pizza stone or heavy baking tray inside the oven. Place the par-baked pizza crust on a piece of baking parchment for easy transfer. Spread the beans all over the par-baked pizza crust, leaving a bit uncovered around the perimeter. Evenly sprinkle both cheeses on top of the beans.

2. Evenly top with the chicken, olives, coriander, tomato, and spring onion.

3. Brush olive oil around the outside edge of the crust. Place the pizza directly on the preheated pizza stone or baking tray. Bake for 12–15 minutes or until the crust is golden brown and the cheese has melted. Slice and serve hot with the desired toppings.

Tip ....
Consider adding red onions, or substituting cooked minced beef for the chicken.

Serves:
8–9

Prep time:
10 minutes

Cook time:
25 minutes

75g (2½oz) salted butter, melted, plus extra for greasing

160g (5¾oz) No. 1 All-Purpose Flour Blend (see p24)

125g (4½oz) American cornmeal, or medium or coarse polenta

1½ tsp xanthan gum

½ tsp salt

1 tsp baking powder

½ tsp bicarbonate of soda

65g (2¼oz) golden granulated sugar

1 large egg

240ml (8fl oz) buttermilk

Nothing goes better with a bowl of chilli or stew than a slice of cornbread. This easy-to-make recipe is moist, sweet, and fluffy straight out of the oven: no butter and honey required (but of course, if you want some, I won't judge).

Cornbread

1. Preheat the oven to 180°C (160°C fan/350°F/Gas 4). Grease the base only of a 20cm (8in) square baking dish. In a large bowl, whisk together the No. 1 All-Purpose Flour Blend, cornmeal, xanthan gum, salt, baking powder, and bicarbonate of soda until thoroughly combined.

2. In a medium bowl, whisk the melted butter with the sugar until thick and smooth. Add the egg and buttermilk and whisk until well combined.

3. Add the wet ingredients to the dry ingredients. Whisk until smooth. Pour the batter into the prepared baking dish and bake for 20–25 minutes or until a toothpick inserted into the centre comes out clean.

4. Cool in the dish for at least 5 minutes before cutting. Serve immediately.

Store it

Store in an airtight container in the refrigerator for up to 5 days, or in the freezer for up to 3 months. Defrost at room temperature, in a microwave, or wrapped in foil in the oven.

Tip

Fold in these optional additions before transferring to the baking dish: 1–2 chopped jalapeños, 100g (3½oz) grated Cheddar cheese, 1 small can chopped green chillies, or 100g (3½oz) bacon lardons.

Makes:
8–10

Prep time:
15 minutes, plus
1 hour to rise

Cook time:
20 minutes

Special equipment:
cooking thermometer

240ml (8fl oz) warm
water at 40–43°C
(105–110°F)

2 tbsp raw honey

560–640g (1¼lb–1lb 7oz)
No. 1 All-Purpose Flour
Blend (see p24), plus up
to 80g (2¾oz) extra as
needed, and
for dusting

7g (¼oz) sachet fast-
action dried yeast

1 tsp xanthan gum

2 tsp salt

½ tsp baking powder

85g (3oz) plain yogurt

1 tbsp apple cider vinegar

1 large egg

avocado oil, or olive oil,
for greasing and
brushing

75g (2½oz) salted butter

3 garlic cloves, finely
chopped or grated

Dipping warm bread in dips or sauces is something I miss terribly when eating out. Indian food is definitely not the same without a piece of naan to soak up the butter chicken or tikka masala sauce. I have been known to sneak in some garlicky gluten-free naan to Indian restaurants, and now you can sneak this recipe in with you, too!

Garlic Butter Naan

1. In a stand mixer fitted with the paddle attachment, or in a large bowl, stir together the warm water and honey until the honey has dissolved.

2. In a medium bowl, whisk together 560g (1¼lb) of the No. 1 All-Purpose Flour Blend, the yeast, xanthan gum, salt, and baking powder. Mix this into the warm honeyed water on low speed.

3. On low speed, add the yogurt, vinegar, and egg. Increase the speed to medium and continue to mix for 2 minutes. The dough will still be sticky but should pull away from the edges of the bowl. If the dough is too sticky and not pulling away from the sides at all, mix in more flour 1 tablespoon at a time until the dough just starts to pull away. Do not add more than 640g (1lb 7oz) in total.

4. Grease a medium bowl with oil, and lightly grease your hands. Remove the dough from the mixing bowl and shape into a ball. Place the ball of dough into the greased bowl. Cover with a damp towel and let rise in a warm place for about 1 hour, or until almost doubled in size.

5. Toward the end of the rise time, prepare the garlic butter. In a small sauté pan over a medium heat, melt the butter. Add the garlic and cook for 1–2 minutes. Remove the pan from the heat, strain, and discard the garlic. Set aside.

6. Once the dough has risen to almost double in size, remove from the bowl and place on a lightly floured surface. Divide the dough into 8–10 pieces (depending on the desired size of the naans). Roll each piece into a ball.

7. Heat a large cast-iron frying pan over a medium-high heat. With a rolling pin, roll out each ball on the lightly floured surface until slightly thinner than 5mm (¼in) thick. Brush both sides with the garlic butter.

8. Working 1 or 2 at a time, add the rolled-out dough to the hot frying pan and cook for 1 minute, or until the dough starts to bubble and the bottom is lightly golden brown. Flip the dough and cook for an additional 30–60 seconds. Transfer the naan to a plate and cover with a sheet of kitchen paper. Repeat with the remaining dough.

9. Keep covered until ready to serve. Serve warm or at room temperature, brushed with any remaining garlic butter.

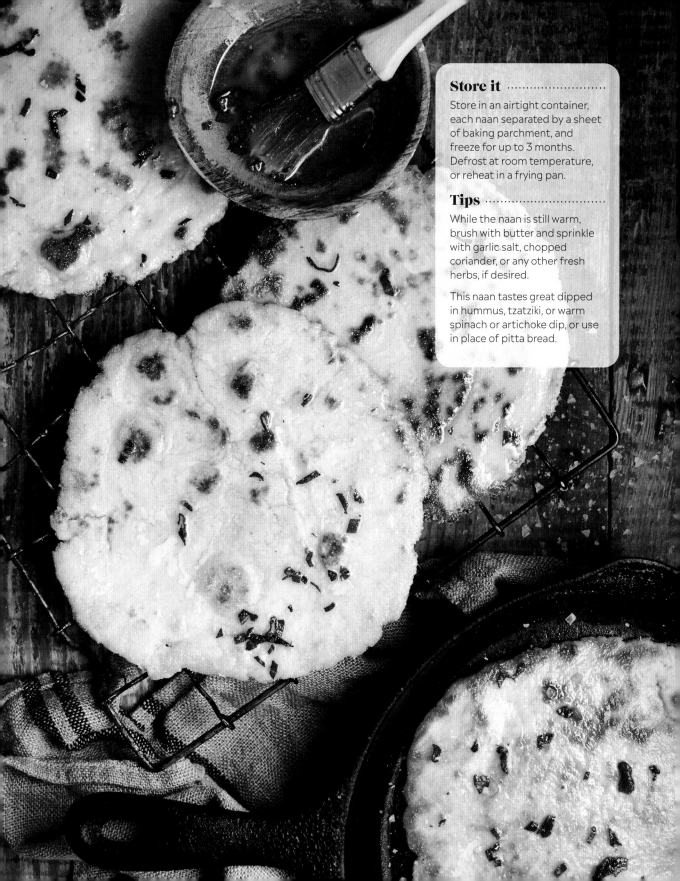

Store it

Store in an airtight container, each naan separated by a sheet of baking parchment, and freeze for up to 3 months. Defrost at room temperature, or reheat in a frying pan.

Tips

While the naan is still warm, brush with butter and sprinkle with garlic salt, chopped coriander, or any other fresh herbs, if desired.

This naan tastes great dipped in hummus, tzatziki, or warm spinach or artichoke dip, or use in place of pitta bread.

Makes:
1 x 23cm (9in) loaf

Prep time:
20 minutes, plus
1½ hours to rise

Cook time:
45 minutes

Special equipment:
cooking thermometer

340g (12oz) Ancient Grain
Flour Blend
(see p24)
80g (2¾oz) No. 1
All-Purpose Flour Blend
(see p24)
1 tsp salt
2 tsp fast-action dried
yeast
2½ tsp xanthan gum
1 large egg, at room
temperature
120ml (4fl oz) whole milk
160ml (5½fl oz) hot water
45g (1½oz) salted butter,
melted
75g (2½oz) raw honey
1 tbsp apple cider vinegar
3 tbsp sesame seeds
(optional)
3 tbsp sunflower seeds
(optional)
3 tbsp pumpkin seeds
(optional), roughly
chopped
cooking spray, for greasing

I could eat a slice of white bread with butter for breakfast, lunch, dinner, and every snack, but every once in a while, I decide a healthier option might be best. This ancient grain bread is soft and moist and tastes just like a slice of white bread, but with the health benefits of ancient grains.

Ancient Grain Sandwich Bread

1. In a medium bowl, whisk together the Ancient Grain Flour Blend, No. 1 All-Purpose Flour Blend, salt, yeast, and xanthan gum.

2. In a stand mixer fitted with the paddle attachment, or in a large bowl, beat the egg for 1 minute on medium-high speed.

3. In a small bowl, combine the milk and the hot water. Once combined, the liquid temperature should be 40–43°C (105–110°F). If it's too hot, let it cool down, and if it's too cold, microwave for a few seconds.

4. Add the warm milk-water mixture, butter, honey, and vinegar to the egg, and beat on medium-high speed until combined.

5. Slowly beat in the flour mixture on low speed. Increase the speed to medium and beat for 3 minutes. The dough will be very sticky, as well as thinner and less pliable than gluten-based dough. If adding sesame seeds, sunflower seeds, and pumpkin seeds, do so now and beat for an additional 1 minute.

6. Lightly spray only the base of a 23 x 12.5cm (9 x 5in) loaf tin with cooking spray. Evenly spread the dough into the loaf pan. If the dough is too sticky to spread with a spatula, wet your fingers and spread with your fingertips.

7. Cover with a greased sheet of baking parchment and set in a warm place to rise for 1–1½ hours or until the dough has risen to the top of the tin.

8. Toward the end of the rise time, preheat the oven to 180°C (160°C fan/ 350°F/Gas 4). Bake for 40–45 minutes. The bread is done when the internal temperature reaches 96–99°C (205–210°F). When it is ready, do not take the bread out of the oven. Turn off the oven and open the oven door. Let the bread slowly cool in the oven for 10–15 minutes before removing it.

9. Remove the bread from the oven and let cool completely on a wire rack in the tin. Remove from the tin, slice, and serve at room temperature or warmed up.

Store it

Once cool, slice the loaf and store in an airtight container, each slice separated by a sheet of baking parchment. Store in the freezer for up to 3 months. Defrost at room temperature, or pop directly into the toaster.

Makes:
1 x 20cm (8in) loaf

Prep time:
20 minutes, plus
1½ hours to rise

Cook time:
45 minutes

Special equipment:
cooking thermometer

480g (1lb 1oz) No. 1
   All-Purpose Flour Blend
   (see p24)

2 tbsp golden granulated
   sugar

1½ tsp salt

2 tsp fast-action dried
   yeast (or active dry
   yeast; see tip, p104)

3 tsp xanthan gum

1 large egg

120ml (4fl oz) whole milk

60ml (5½fl oz) hot water

60g (2oz) salted butter,
   melted

1 tbsp raw honey

1 tbsp apple cider vinegar

vegetable oil or light
   cooking spray,
   for greasing

As soon as someone finds out I'm a gluten-free baker, their first question is: "Do you have a white bread recipe?" A good gluten-free white bread is almost impossible to find in a store; they're usually crumbly and cardboard-like. This recipe is moist, soft, and will have you guessing whether or not it is really gluten-free.

Easy White Sandwich Bread

1. In a medium bowl, whisk together the No. 1 All-Purpose Flour Blend, sugar, salt, yeast, and xanthan gum.

2. In a stand mixer fitted with the paddle attachment, or in a large bowl, beat the egg for 1 minute on medium-high speed.

3. In a small bowl, combine the milk and the hot water. Once combined, the liquid temperature should be 40–43°C (105–110°F). If it's too hot, let it cool down, and if it's too cold, microwave for a few seconds.

4. Add the warm milk-water mixture, butter, honey, and vinegar to the egg, and beat on low speed until combined. Slowly beat in the flour mixture on low speed. Increase the speed to medium and beat for 3 minutes.

5. Evenly spread the dough into an ungreased 20 x 12.5cm (8 x 5in) loaf tin. Cover with a greased sheet of baking parchment and set in a warm place to rise for 1–1½ hours or until the dough has risen to the top of the tin.

6. Toward the end of the rise time, preheat the oven to 180°C (160°C fan/ 350°F/Gas 4). Bake for 40–45 minutes. The bread is done when the internal temperature reaches 96–99°C (205–210°F).

7. When it is ready, do not take the bread out of the oven. Turn off the oven and open the door. Let the bread slowly cool in the oven for 10–15 minutes before removing it.

8. Take the bread out of the oven and let cool completely on a wire rack in the tin. Remove from the tin, slice, and serve at room temperature or warmed up.

Store it

Once cool, slice the loaf and store in an airtight container, each slice separated by a sheet of baking parchment. Store in the freezer for up to 3 months. Defrost at room temperature, or pop directly into the toaster.

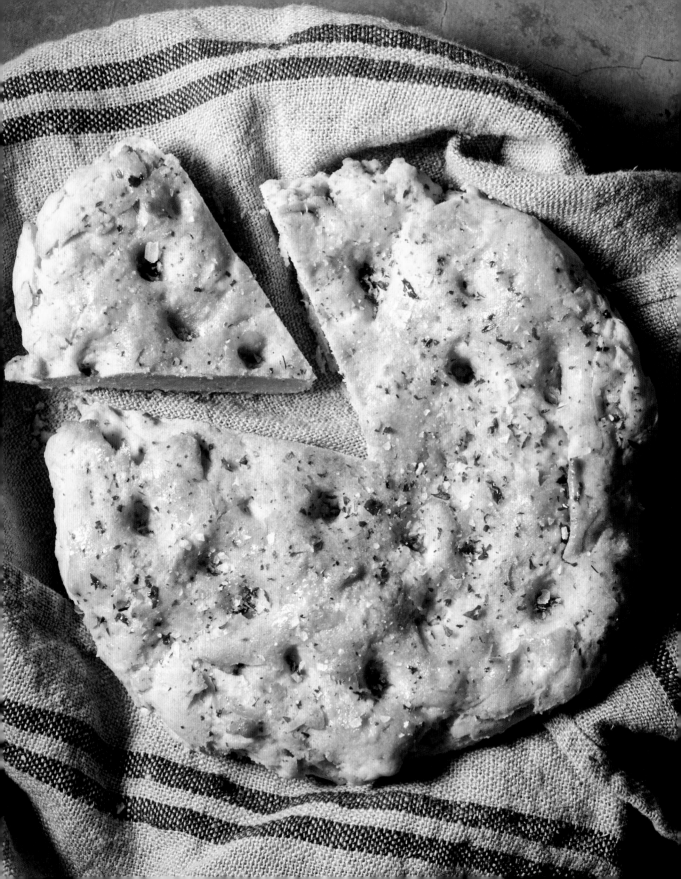

Makes:
1 x 23cm (9in) loaf

Prep time:
20 minutes, plus
1 hour to rise

Cook time:
25 minutes

Special equipment:
cooking thermometer

2 tbsp olive oil, plus extra
for greasing
320g (11oz) No. 1
All-Purpose Flour Blend
(see p24)
1 tsp xanthan gum
1 tsp salt
1 tbsp golden granulated
sugar
7g (¼oz) sachet fast-
action dried yeast
½ tsp dried thyme
¼ tsp onion powder
¼ tsp garlic powder
½ tsp dried basil
½ tsp dried oregano
1 large egg, at room
temperature
180ml (6fl oz) warm
water, at 40-43°C
(105-110°F)
2 tsp apple cider vinegar
chopped fresh herbs, such
as basil, oregano, or
parsley, or garlic salt
(optional), to top

I love the fluffy texture of focaccia bread, so I set out to create a version that is as good as its gluten-packed counterpart. My oldest son is a picky eater, and the first time I made this recipe, he ate the entire loaf himself. The olive oil and seasonings give it great flavour, and it has just the right crispiness on the outside and fluffiness on the inside.

Focaccia

1. Generously grease only the base of a 23cm (9in) round or square springform or cake tin with oil.

2. In a medium bowl, stir together the No. 1 All-Purpose Flour Blend, xanthan gum, salt, sugar, yeast, thyme, onion powder, garlic powder, basil, and oregano.

3. In a stand mixer fitted with the paddle attachment, or in a large bowl, beat the egg for 30 seconds on high speed. Briefly incorporate the warm water, vinegar, and oil.

4. On low speed, carefully add the flour mixture to the wet ingredients. Scrape down the sides and increase the speed to medium-high. Beat for 2 minutes.

5. Pour the dough into the prepared tin; it will be very sticky. Wet your fingertips with warm water and gently spread the dough evenly in the pan. Very gently create dimples on the top with your fingers, if desired.

6. Cover with baking parchment and set in a warm place to rise. Let the dough rise for 30 minutes to 1 hour or until doubled in size. Do not let the dough rise more than double, or it will fall flat when baked. When the dough has almost completed its rise, preheat the oven to 200°C (180°C fan/400°F/Gas 6).

7. Gently spray or brush the top of the risen dough with oil (be careful not to deflate the dough) and sprinkle with herbs, or garlic salt, if desired.

8. Bake for 20–25 minutes or until golden brown. When ready, do not take it out of the oven. Turn off the oven and open the oven door. Let the bread slowly cool in the oven for 10–15 minutes before removing it. Slice and serve warm.

Store it
This bread is best eaten fresh, but store leftovers in an airtight container for up to 2 days. Warm it in the oven or microwave to soften it up. You can also store in an airtight container in the freezer for up to 3 months and defrost at room temperature.

Tips
Be sure the egg is at room temperature and that your water is the correct temperature. If the ingredients are too cold, the yeast will not activate and create a proper rise.

Wet your fingers with warm water when spreading out the dough, to avoid damaging the rise.

Allowing the bread to cool slowly helps prevent your loaf from sinking after it's baked.

Makes:
8

Prep time:
30 minutes, plus
1 hour to rise

Cook time:
20 minutes

Special equipment:
cooking thermometer

480g (1lb 1oz) No. 1
All-Purpose Flour Blend
(see p24)
60g (2oz) sweet sorghum
flour
1 tbsp fast-action dried
yeast
1½ tsp salt
3 tbsp golden granulated
sugar
2 tsp xanthan gum
180ml (6fl oz) sparkling
water
120ml (4fl oz) hot water
70g (2¼oz) salted butter,
softened
2 large eggs
2 tsp apple cider vinegar
vegetable oil, if needed

*I get so tired of having my burger "lettuce wrapped"; while that may
be low carb-friendly, a burger is just not a burger without a bun. Many
of the gluten-free hamburger buns you can buy crumble and fall apart
once a juicy patty is added. My hamburger bun recipe is so tasty you
will feel like you are enjoying a real burger again!*

Hamburger Buns

1. Line 2 baking trays with baking parchment. In a stand mixer fitted with the paddle attachment, or in a large bowl, whisk together the No. 1 All-Purpose Flour Blend, sorghum flour, yeast, salt, sugar, and xanthan gum.

2. In a small bowl, add the sparkling water to the hot water. Once combined, the liquid temperature should be 40–43°C (105–110°F). If it's too hot, let it cool down, and if it's too cold, microwave for a few seconds.

3. Add the water, 30g (1oz) of the butter, the eggs, and vinegar to the flour mixture. Start mixing on low speed, and gradually increase the speed to medium. Mix for 2 minutes.

4. Divide the dough into 8 equal pieces. Shape each piece into a ball and place on the prepared baking trays. If the dough is too sticky to work with, rub oil on your hands before rolling.

5. Flatten the balls into 7.5cm (3in) discs, cover, and let rise for about 1 hour, or until nearly doubled in size.

6. Preheat the oven to 190°C (170°C fan/375°F/Gas 5). Melt the remaining butter. Brush half the butter on the buns. Bake for 15–18 minutes or until golden brown.

7. Remove the buns from the oven and brush with the remaining melted butter. Cool the buns on a wire rack. Once cooled, slice and serve.

Store it

Store the sliced buns in an airtight container in the freezer for up to 3 months.
To defrost, wrap in kitchen paper and microwave for 30 seconds, or defrost at
room temperature.

Tip

Brush with butter and grill or toast before using.

Makes:
8 x 15–17.5cm (6–7in)
tortillas

Prep time:
30 minutes

Cook time:
25 minutes

320g (11oz) No. 1
   All-Purpose Flour Blend
   (see p24)
30g (1oz) tapioca flour,
   plus extra for dusting
1 tsp salt
¼ tsp baking powder
1 tbsp golden granulated
   sugar
½ tsp xanthan gum
2 tbsp white vegetable fat
1 tsp apple cider vinegar
180ml (6fl oz) ice-cold
   water

A soft, mild, gluten-free flour tortilla is difficult to find, and corn tortillas get boring. Store-bought gluten-free flour tortillas have come a long way, but I'm yet to find one I like without processed ingredients. These home-made tortillas have just a few ingredients and are even Max-approved, so my son can enjoy his favourite quesadillas!

Flour Tortillas

1. In a stand mixer fitted with the paddle attachment, or in a large bowl, whisk together the No. 1 All-Purpose Flour Blend, tapioca flour, salt, baking powder, sugar, and xanthan gum.

2. Add the vegetable fat. Mix on medium-high speed until the fat is well dispersed and pea-sized crumbs have formed.

3. On low speed, add the vinegar and water. Increase the speed to medium and mix for 2 minutes.

4. Heat a cast-iron frying pan or griddle pan over medium heat. Place the dough on a piece of baking parchment and divide into 8 equal pieces. Roll each piece into a ball. Place a damp sheet of kitchen paper over the balls of dough until ready to use.

5. Place a ball of dough between 2 sheets of baking parchment and roll out into a 15–17.5cm (6–7in) circle. If the dough begins to stick, dust a small amount of tapioca flour onto the baking parchment and dough.

6. Carefully transfer the rolled-out dough to the hot pan. Cook for 1½ minutes, flip, and cook for an additional 1½ minutes. Transfer to a plate lined with a damp sheet of kitchen paper and cover with another damp sheet of kitchen paper. Continue to cook the remaining tortillas, placing a damp sheet of kitchen paper between each.

7. Once all of the tortillas have been cooked, serve immediately.

Store it

Store in an airtight container, each tortilla separated by a sheet of baking parchment, and freeze for up to 3 months. To defrost, one at a time, place a tortilla between sheets of damp kitchen paper and microwave for 20 seconds.

Tips

Placing the freshly cooked tortillas between damp sheets of kitchen paper helps them to stay soft and flexible. However, if you leave them for too long, the paper will begin to stick to the tortillas. To avoid this, remove the tortillas from the papers before they are completely cooled.

This recipe works brilliantly with a tortilla press, for perfectly round and perfectly cooked tortillas.

Sweet Loaves, Muffins, & Scones

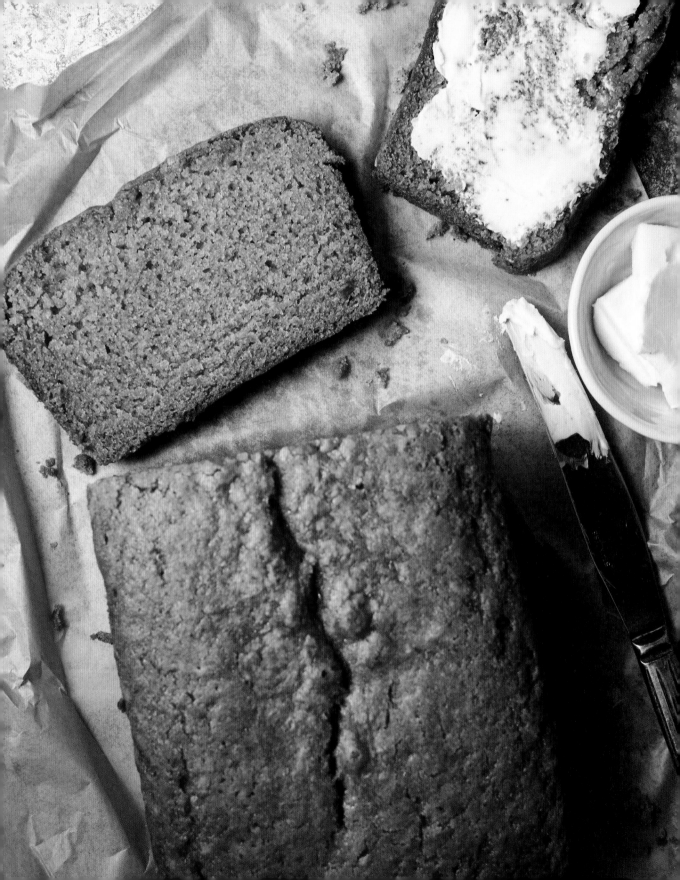

Makes:
1 x 23cm (9in) loaf

Prep time:
15 minutes

Cook time:
1 hour

I have this recipe to thank for starting my gluten-free baking craze and making me famous for gluten-free baked goods in my home town. In the process of recreating my mum's Thanksgiving cake, the recipe turned into loaves of pumpkin bread. Before I knew it, I was selling it to shops around town. Once you try this, you'll know why.

The Pumpkin Bread That Started It All

300g (10oz) golden
granulated sugar

140ml (4¾fl oz) light
vegetable oil, such as
avocado oil

2 large eggs

225g (8oz) canned 100
per cent pure pumpkin

½ tsp salt

1 tsp xanthan gum

1 tsp baking powder

½ tsp bicarbonate of soda

½ tsp ground cinnamon

¼ tsp ground allspice

¼ tsp ground nutmeg

⅛ tsp ground cloves

280g (9½oz) No. 1
All-Purpose Flour Blend
(see p24)

80ml (2½fl oz) water

butter, to serve (optional)

1. Preheat the oven to 170°C (150°C fan/325°F/Gas 3½). In a stand mixer fitted with the whisk attachment, or in a large bowl, whisk together the sugar and oil on medium speed. Add the eggs and whisk on medium-high speed until well combined. Add the pumpkin and whisk until well incorporated.

2. In a separate medium bowl, whisk together the salt, xanthan gum, baking powder, bicarbonate of soda, cinnamon, allspice, nutmeg, cloves, and No. 1 All-Purpose Flour Blend.

3. Stir alternate batches of the dry ingredients and the water into the pumpkin mixture, starting and ending with the flour mix. Stir until well combined.

4. Pour the batter into an ungreased 23 x 12.5cm (9 x 5in) loaf tin and bake for 1 hour, or until a toothpick inserted into the centre comes out clean. Cool completely before slicing and serving with butter for spreading, if you like.

Store it ···

Store in an airtight container for up to 3 days, or freeze for up to 3 months. Either freeze the whole loaf, or freeze slices individually. Defrost at room temperature.

Tip ···

This bread makes an incredible dessert for autumn if you spread a layer of Cream Cheese Frosting (see p160) on top.

Makes:
1 x 23cm (9in) loaf

Prep time:
15 minutes

Cook time:
1½ hours

75ml (2½fl oz) light vegetable oil, such as avocado oil, plus extra for greasing

275g (9½oz) No. 1 All-Purpose Flour Blend, or Ancient Grain Flour Blend (see p24)

1 tsp bicarbonate of soda

1 tsp xanthan gum

¼ tsp ground cinnamon

½ tsp salt

200g (7oz) golden granulated sugar

2 large eggs, at room temperature

3 very ripe small bananas, mashed

2 tbsp sour cream

1 tsp vanilla extract

60g (2oz) chopped pecans

butter, to serve (optional)

After my pumpkin bread became a hit at the local farmer's market, I wanted to expand my bread offerings. This banana nut bread is the second gluten-free bread recipe I ever created, and probably my husband's favourite when served warm with butter. Serve this to family and friends, and no one will ever know it's gluten-free.

Banana Nut Bread

1. Preheat the oven to 180°C (160°C fan/350°F/Gas 4) and grease only the base of a 23 x 12.5cm (9 x 5in) loaf tin. In a small bowl, whisk together the No. 1 All-Purpose Flour Blend, bicarbonate of soda, xanthan gum, cinnamon, and salt.

2. In a stand mixer fitted with the paddle attachment, or in a large bowl, beat the sugar and eggs on medium-low speed for about 3 minutes, until light in colour.

3. While on low speed, slowly drizzle the oil into the sugar-egg mixture, and then increase the speed to medium and beat until well combined.

4. Add the mashed bananas, sour cream, and vanilla into the wet ingredients, and beat on low speed until just combined.

5. Gently stir the dry ingredients into the wet ingredients, being careful not to overmix. Gently stir in the chopped pecans. Pour the batter into the loaf tin. Bake for 50–60 minutes or until a toothpick inserted into the centre comes out clean. (If using the Ancient Grain Flour Blend, you may need to add 10–20 minutes to the baking time.)

6. Let cool in the tin for 10 minutes, and then transfer to a wire rack to cool completely, or slice and serve warm with butter, if you like.

Store it

Store in an airtight container for up to 3 days, or freeze for up to 3 months. Either freeze the whole loaf, or freeze slices individually. Defrost at room temperature.

Makes:
2 x 23cm (9in) loaves

Prep time:
15 minutes

Cook time:
1 hour

100g (3½oz) white vegetable fat, plus extra for greasing

225g (8oz) fresh cranberries (or frozen cranberries, defrosted)

400g (14oz) golden granulated sugar

225g (8oz) cream cheese, softened

3 large eggs

1½ tsp vanilla extract

1 tsp apple cider vinegar

320g (11oz) No. 1 All-Purpose Flour Blend (see p24)

2 tsp xanthan gum

1 tsp baking powder

½ tsp bicarbonate of soda

½ tsp salt

¼ tsp ground mace

My mum used to make cranberry bread every Christmas and give it to neighbours as presents. It felt like Christmas-time the second I could smell or taste it. This gluten-free rendition is so amazing when warmed up and slathered with butter.

Christmas Cranberry Bread

1. Preheat the oven to 180°C (160°C fan/350°F/Gas 4) and lightly grease only the bases of two 23 x 12.5cm (9 x 5in) loaf tins. In a food processor, pulse the cranberries until coarsely chopped. In a small bowl, stir the cranberries with half the sugar.

2. In a stand mixer fitted with the paddle attachment, or in large bowl, beat the cream cheese, vegetable fat, and the remaining sugar until well combined.

3. Starting on low speed, beat in the eggs one at a time, and then increase the speed to high and beat in the vanilla and vinegar.

4. In a large bowl, whisk together the No. 1 All-Purpose Flour Blend, xanthan gum, baking powder, bicarbonate of soda, salt, and mace until combined.

5. Pour the flour mixture into the wet ingredients and mix on low speed until combined. Gently stir in the sugared cranberries.

6. Pour the batter into the 2 loaf tins and bake for 50–60 minutes or until a toothpick inserted into the centres comes out clean.

7. Cool for 10 minutes in the tins and then transfer to a wire rack to cool completely. Slice and serve.

Store it

Store in an airtight container for up to 3 days, or freeze for up to 3 months. Either freeze the whole loaf, or freeze slices individually. Defrost at room temperature.

Makes:
1 x 23cm (9in) loaf

Prep time:
20 minutes

Cook time:
1 hour

60g (2oz) salted butter, melted and cooled, plus extra for greasing

320g (11oz) No. 1 All-Purpose Flour Blend (see p24)

200g (7oz) golden granulated sugar

1 tbsp baking powder

1½ tsp xanthan gum

½ tsp salt

80ml (2½fl oz) sour cream

120ml (4fl oz) whole milk

2 large eggs

butter, to serve (optional)

For the swirl

45g (1½oz) light brown sugar

1 tsp ground cinnamon

30g (1oz) chopped walnuts or pecans

For the glaze

30g (1oz) icing sugar

1 tbsp whole milk

½ tbsp light vegetable oil, such as avocado oil

¼ tsp vanilla extract

If you love cinnamon rolls, then you will love this quick bread recipe. You dump all the ingredients into one bowl and then beat the mixture. Easy peasy to make and very little washing up!

Cinnamon Swirl Bread

1. Preheat the oven to 180°C (160°C fan/350°F/Gas 4) and lightly grease only the base of a 23 x 12.5cm (9 x 5in) loaf tin.

2. Prepare the cinnamon swirl. In a small bowl, stir together the brown sugar, cinnamon, and chopped nuts. Set aside.

3. In a stand mixer fitted with the paddle attachment, or in a large bowl, combine the No. 1 All-Purpose Flour Blend, golden granulated sugar, baking powder, xanthan gum, salt, sour cream, melted butter, milk, and eggs. Beat the mixture on low speed for 1 minute. Scrape down the sides of the bowl and beat on medium speed for 1 minute longer.

4. Pour one-third of the batter into the loaf tin. (The batter will be very thick and you will need to use your fingers to spread it in the tin.) Sprinkle half the cinnamon swirl over the batter. Pour another one-third of the batter into the tin, spreading with your fingers, and sprinkle with the remaining cinnamon swirl. Pour in the remaining batter and spread evenly.

5. Using a skewer or long toothpick, gently cut through the batter to swirl the cinnamon swirl around. Bake for 45 minutes. Cover the loaf with foil and bake for an additional 15 minutes, or until a toothpick inserted into the centre comes out clean.

6. Pour the glaze over the hot bread while it is still in the tin. Let cool completely in the tin before slicing. Serve the slices at room temperature, or warm them up and serve with butter.

   Glaze: In a small bowl, stir together the icing sugar, milk, oil, and vanilla.

Store it ···

Store in an airtight container for up to 3 days, or freeze the slices individually wrapped for up to 3 months. Defrost at room temperature.

Makes:
16–18

Prep time:
20 minutes

Cook time:
25 minutes

These are the only muffins my son Max will ever eat. They taste just like snickerdoodle cookies – which are cookies with their edges rolled in cinnamon sugar – and are light and fluffy. I love to serve these to my kids as dessert, especially with butter for spreading.

Max's Snickerdoodle Muffins

225g (8oz) salted butter, softened, plus extra for greasing
360g (13oz) No. 2 All-Purpose Flour Blend (see p24)
1½ tsp xanthan gum
½ tsp ground cinnamon
½ tsp salt
¾ tsp baking powder
¾ tsp bicarbonate of soda
¾ tsp cream of tartar
200g (7oz) golden granulated sugar
2 large eggs, at room temperature
1 tsp apple cider vinegar
2 tsp vanilla extract
240ml (8fl oz) sour cream

For the topping
60g (2oz) golden granulated sugar
3 tbsp light brown sugar
1 tsp ground cinnamon
40g (1½oz) salted butter, melted

1. Preheat the oven to 180°C (160°C fan/350°F/Gas 4) and lightly grease the muffin tins (do not use paper cases). In a large bowl, whisk together the No. 2 All-Purpose Flour Blend, xanthan gum, cinnamon, salt, baking powder, bicarbonate of soda, and cream of tartar.

2. In a stand mixer fitted with the paddle attachment, or in a large bowl, cream the butter and sugar on high speed for 3 minutes or until light and fluffy.

3. Add the eggs one at a time, beating on medium-high speed for 30 seconds between each addition. Add the vinegar, vanilla, and sour cream, and beat on medium-low speed until combined, scraping down the sides as necessary.

4. Add the wet ingredients to the flour mixture and stir just until combined; the batter will be thick. Using an ice-cream scoop, fill each muffin mould about two-thirds full. Bake for 25 minutes, or until the muffins spring back when lightly touched and a toothpick inserted into the centres comes out clean.

5. While the muffins are baking, in a small bowl, make the topping. Stir together the granulated sugar, brown sugar, and cinnamon until well combined.

6. Remove the muffins from the oven when they're ready and leave in the tins until cool enough to touch. While the muffins are still warm, working one at a time, lightly brush the top of each muffin with butter and roll in the cinnamon-sugar mixture. Cool completely on a wire rack before serving.

Store it
Store in an airtight container in the refrigerator for up to 1 week, or freeze for up to 3 months. Defrost at room temperature, or reheat in the microwave.

Tip
A silicone muffin mould makes it very easy to pop these muffins out.

Makes:
14

Prep time:
20 minutes, plus cooling

Cook time:
30 minutes

320g (11oz) No. 1
  All-Purpose Flour Blend
  (see p24), plus 1 tbsp
  for dusting
200g (7oz) golden
  granulated sugar
½ tsp salt
2 tsp baking powder
2 tsp xanthan gum
2 large eggs
75ml (2½fl oz) light
  vegetable oil, such as
  avocado oil
1 tsp apple cider vinegar
120ml (4fl oz) whole milk
120ml (4fl oz) sour cream
150g (5½oz) fresh or
  frozen blueberries

For the topping

85g (3oz) light brown
  sugar
80g (2¾oz) No. 1
  All-Purpose Flour Blend
  (see p24)
½ tsp xanthan gum
¼ tsp salt
¼ tsp ground cinnamon
40g (1½oz) salted butter,
  chilled, cut into
  small pieces

These muffins are so soft and moist that no one will ever know they are gluten-free. The crumb topping gives them the perfect amount of sweetness. Adding a touch of butter to your warm blueberry muffins when you eat these makes them unbelievably scrumptious.

Blueberry Muffins

1. Preheat the oven to 190°C (170°C fan/375°F/Gas 5) and line the muffin tins with paper cases. Prepare the topping. In a medium bowl, stir together the brown sugar, the 80g (2¾oz) of No. 1 All-Purpose Flour Blend, xanthan gum, salt, and cinnamon. Cut in the butter with a pastry cutter or a fork until pea-sized crumbs are formed. Squeeze the mixture together with your hands and then break it up to form crumbs again. Set aside.

2. In a large bowl, stir together the 320g (11¼oz) of No. 1 All-Purpose Flour Blend, the sugar, salt, baking powder, and xanthan gum until combined.

3. In a separate medium bowl, whisk the eggs, oil, vinegar, and milk until combined. Stir the wet ingredients into the dry ingredients just until combined, being careful not to overmix.

4. Gently stir in the sour cream. Toss the blueberries with the remaining 1 tablespoon No. 1 All-Purpose Flour Blend before mixing in; this will prevent them from sinking to the bottom. Fold in the blueberries.

5. Using an ice-cream scoop, fill each muffin case about two-thirds full. Top the muffins evenly with the crumb topping. Bake for 28–30 minutes or until a toothpick inserted into the centres comes out clean. Let cool in the tins for 5 minutes. Serve warm.

Store it ....

Store in an airtight container in the refrigerator for up to 5 days, or in the freezer for up to 3 months. Defrost at room temperature, or reheat in the microwave.

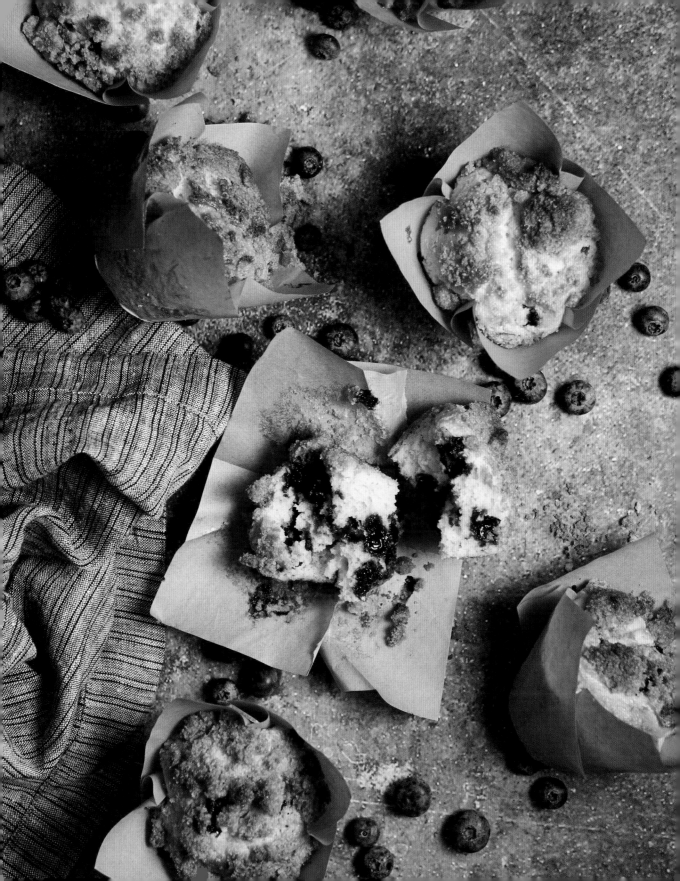

Makes:
12

Prep time:
20 minutes, plus cooling

Cook time:
30 minutes

200g (7oz) No. 1
   All-Purpose Flour Blend
   (see p24)
45g (1½oz) light brown
   sugar, or coconut sugar
70g (2¼oz) golden
   granulated sugar
1 tsp ground cinnamon
1½ tsp baking powder
¼ tsp salt
1 tsp xanthan gum
50g (1¾oz) rolled oats
   (certified gluten-free)
2 large eggs
40g (1½oz) salted butter,
   melted
1 tsp vanilla extract
1 tsp apple cider vinegar
120ml (4fl oz) sour cream
2 tbsp pure maple syrup
125g (4½oz) grated
   courgette
60g (2oz) grated carrot
4 tbsp demerara sugar
butter, to serve (optional)

Need to sneak some additional vegetables into your children's diet? These muffins give you a yummy, if sneaky, way to do just that, without them noticing. These are a great school or work day breakfast, when everyone is in a hurry.

Carrot Courgette Muffins

1. Preheat the oven to 180°C (160°C fan/350°F/Gas 4) and line the muffin tin with paper cases. In a large bowl, stir together the No. 1 All-Purpose Flour Blend, brown sugar, golden granulated sugar, cinnamon, baking powder, salt, and xanthan gum until well combined. Stir in the oats.

2. In a separate medium bowl, whisk together the eggs, melted butter, vanilla, vinegar, sour cream, and syrup. Add the wet ingredients to the dry ingredients, and stir until just combined, being careful not to overmix. The batter will be thick and lumpy.

3. Add the courgette and carrot, and stir until just incorporated. Using an ice-cream scoop, fill each muffin case about two-thirds full.

4. Bake for 25–30 minutes or until a toothpick inserted into the centres comes out clean. Cool in the tin for 5 minutes, and then transfer to a wire rack to cool completely, or serve warm with butter.

Store it

Store in an airtight container in the refrigerator for up to 3 days, or in the freezer for up to 3 months. Defrost at room temperature, or reheat in the microwave.

Makes:
about 24

Prep time:
30 minutes, plus cooling

Cook time:
35 minutes

115g (4oz) canned
crushed pineapple

200g (7oz) coconut sugar

100g (3½oz) Ancient
Grain Flour Blend
(see p24)

120g (4½oz)No. 1
All-Purpose Flour Blend
(see p24)

2 tsp ground cinnamon

100g (3½oz) rolled oats
(certified gluten-free)

2 tsp xanthan gum

2 tsp bicarbonate of soda

½ tsp salt

50g (1¾oz) desiccated
coconut

85g (3oz) finely chopped
dried apricots
(unsulphured or
organic)

1 apple, peeled and grated

225g (8oz) grated carrot

50g (1¾oz) chopped
pecans

3 large eggs

1 tsp apple cider vinegar

240ml (8fl oz) sour cream

1 tsp vanilla extract

85g (3oz) pure maple
syrup

demerara sugar, or
coconut sugar,
for topping

butter, to serve (optional)

These muffins are full of fruits and vegetables, making them substantial enough to start your day, plus they're not very sweet. They will definitely fill your tummy. This recipe gets its name from the café where it originated: Morning Glory in Nantucket. These will make your morning glorious, too!

Morning Glory Muffins

1. Place the pineapple in a sieve placed over a bowl to drain very well. Set aside until ready to use. Preheat the oven to 180°C (160°C fan/350°F/Gas 4) and line the muffin tins with paper cases.

2. In a large bowl, whisk together the coconut sugar, Ancient Grain Flour Blend, No. 1 All-Purpose Flour Blend, cinnamon, oats, xanthan gum, bicarbonate of soda, and salt.

3. Add the coconut, apricots, apple, carrot, pecans, and drained crushed pineapple. Stir to mix.

4. In a separate medium bowl, beat the eggs. Add the vinegar, sour cream, vanilla, and maple syrup, and beat until well combined. Pour the wet ingredients into the dry ingredients and stir until combined.

5. Using an ice-cream scoop, fill each muffin case about two-thirds full. Sprinkle demerara sugar or coconut sugar on top. Bake for 30–35 minutes or until a toothpick inserted into the centres comes out clean.

6. Cool in the tins for 5–10 minutes, and then transfer to a wire rack to cool completely, or serve warm with butter.

Store it

Store in an airtight container for up to 3 days, or in the freezer for up to 3 months. Defrost at room temperature, or reheat in the microwave.

Makes:
12

Prep time:
20 minutes, plus cooling

Cook time:
30 minutes

These are my favourite muffins! You'll definitely impress your gluten-eating friends with these. They're great for breakfast, but also sweet enough for dessert. You can bake this recipe as a loaf cake, though the muffins are easier to eat on the run.

Grab 'n' Go Cinnamon Streusel Muffins

280g (9½oz) No. 1 All-Purpose Flour Blend (see p24)

1½ tsp xanthan gum

2 tsp baking powder

1 tsp bicarbonate of soda

115g (4oz) salted butter, softened

100g (3½oz) golden granulated sugar

85g (3oz) light brown sugar

240ml (8fl oz) sour cream

1 tsp apple cider vinegar

1 tsp vanilla extract

2 large eggs

butter, to serve (optional)

For the filling

3 tbsp light brown sugar

3 tbsp No. 1 All-Purpose Flour Blend (see p24)

½ tsp ground cinnamon

For the topping

45g (1½oz) light brown sugar

40g (1½oz) No. 1 All-Purpose Flour Blend (see p24)

¼ tsp xanthan gum

¼ tsp ground cinnamon

20g (¾oz) salted butter, chilled, cut into small pieces

1. Preheat the oven to 180°C (160°C fan/350°F/Gas 4) and line the muffin tin with paper cases. Prepare the filling. In a small bowl, stir together the brown sugar, No. 1 All-Purpose Flour Blend, and cinnamon. Set aside.

2. Prepare the topping. In a small bowl, stir together the brown sugar, No. 1 All-Purpose Flour Blend, xanthan gum, and cinnamon. Using a pastry cutter or fork, cut in the butter until coarse crumbs are formed. Refrigerate until ready to use.

3. For the muffins, in a small bowl, whisk together the No. 1 All-Purpose Flour Blend, xanthan gum, baking powder, and bicarbonate of soda. In a stand mixer fitted with the paddle attachment, or in a large bowl, beat the butter, golden granulated sugar, and brown sugar on high speed until well combined. Add the sour cream, vinegar, and vanilla, and beat on high speed for about 2 minutes.

4. Add the eggs one at a time, beating on high speed after each addition. On low speed, slowly beat the flour mixture into the butter mixture until combined.

5. The batter will be thick and you will need to use wet fingers if you need to spread it out. Place 1 tablespoon of batter into each paper case. Top with ½ tablespoon of cinnamon filling. Add 2 tablespoons more batter on top of each muffin. Top each muffin with 1 tablespoon of crumb topping.

6. Bake for 30 minutes, or until a toothpick inserted into the centres comes out clean and the muffins spring back when touched. Cool in the tin for 5 minutes before removing. Serve warm or at room temperature with butter, if you like.

Loaf Cake: Grease and lightly flour the base of a 20cm (8in) square baking tin. Pour half the batter into the prepared tin. Evenly sprinkle the cinnamon filling on top. Pour the remaining batter on top of the cinnamon filling. Evenly sprinkle the crumb topping mixture over the batter. Bake for 55–60 minutes or until a toothpick inserted into the centre comes out clean.

Store it ···

Store in an airtight container in the refrigerator for up to 5 days, or in the freezer for up to 3 months. Defrost at room temperature, or reheat in the microwave.

Makes:
16

Prep time:
15 minutes, plus cooling

Cook time:
25 minutes

320g (11oz) No. 1 All-Purpose Flour Blend (see p24), plus extra for dusting

2 tsp xanthan gum

4 tbsp golden granulated sugar

1 tbsp baking powder

¾ tsp salt

85g (3oz) white vegetable fat (see tip, below)

2 large eggs

80ml (2½fl oz) canned coconut cream, or double cream, plus extra for brushing

1 tsp vanilla extract

1 tsp raw apple cider vinegar

Icing (see p36, step 8), for coating

My mum came to me and told me that she desperately missed little vanilla scones from the coffee shop after going gluten-free, and she asked me to create a gluten-free version for her. So, here it is. She says that these mini scones taste almost exactly the same.

Little Vanilla Scones

1. Place the oven shelf in the centre of the oven and preheat it to 200°C (180°C fan/400°F/Gas 6). Line a baking tray with baking parchment. In a large bowl, whisk together the No. 1 All-Purpose Flour Blend, xanthan gum, sugar, baking powder, and salt.

2. Using a pastry cutter or fork, cut in the vegetable fat until pea-sized crumbs are formed.

3. In a separate medium bowl, lightly beat the eggs. Then beat in the coconut cream or double cream, vanilla, and vinegar.

4. Make a well in the centre of the dry ingredients and pour the cream mixture into the well. Stir carefully until just combined.

5. Turn the dough out onto a piece of baking parchment or a lightly floured surface. The dough will be very crumbly and will seem too dry; do not be tempted to add extra liquid. Gently knead the dough a few times until it is well mixed and sticks together.

6. Form the dough into a 15cm (6in) square, 2.5–3cm (1–1¼in) thick. Dip a knife into some flour, and then cut the dough into 4 smaller squares. Cut the squares in half diagonally to form 8 triangles. Cut the 8 triangles in half to create 16 mini triangles. Arrange the triangles on the prepared baking tray.

7. Brush the top of each scone with coconut cream or double cream. Bake for 20–25 minutes, or until the tops are golden brown. Cool on a wire rack. Once the scones have cooled, dip them in the icing and let dry completely on a wire rack before serving.

Store it
Let the iced scones cool completely. Store in an airtight container for up to 3 days, or individually wrapped in the freezer for up to 3 months. Defrost at room temperature, or reheat in the oven or microwave.

Tips
This scone is a great base for other flavours. You can add chocolate chips, nuts, or dried fruit, or you can change up the flavour of the icing by using citrus juice instead of water.

If you use a brand of vegetable fat that contains a lot of water, you may find your scones spreading excessively. Chill the dough for at least 1 hour before baking, to help prevent the spreading.

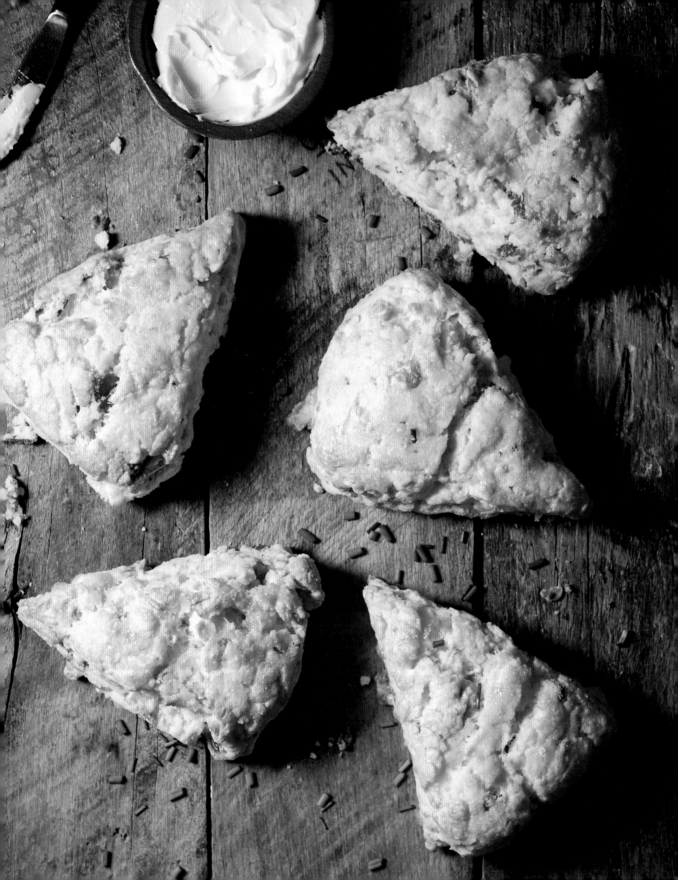

Makes:
8

Prep time:
30 minutes, plus cooling

Cook time:
25 minutes

320g (11oz) No. 1
   All-Purpose Flour Blend
   (see p24), plus extra
   for dusting

2 tsp xanthan gum

2 tbsp golden granulated
   sugar

1 tbsp baking powder

¾ tsp salt

85g (3oz) white vegetable
   fat (see tip, below)

50g (1¾oz) prosciutto,
   chopped

60g (2oz) Gruyère cheese,
   grated

30g (1oz) Parmesan
   cheese, grated

15g (½oz) chopped chives

3 large eggs

120ml (4fl oz) buttermilk

1 tsp apple cider vinegar

1 tbsp water

butter, to serve (optional)

These savoury scones are a great alternative to a bread roll or garlic bread with your meal, or with soup. The prosciutto and chives punch up the flavour, and the Gruyère gives it a perfect cheesy richness.

Gruyère, Prosciutto, & Chive Scones

1. Preheat the oven to 200°C (180°C fan/400°F/Gas 6) and line a baking tray with baking parchment. In a large bowl, whisk together the No. 1 All-Purpose Flour Blend, xanthan gum, sugar, baking powder, and salt.

2. Using a pastry cutter or fork, cut in the vegetable fat until pea-sized crumbs are formed. Stir in the prosciutto, Gruyère, Parmesan, and chives.

3. In a separate small bowl, lightly beat 2 of the eggs, and then beat in the buttermilk and vinegar. Make a well in the centre of the dry ingredients and pour in the egg mixture. Stir until just combined.

4. Turn the dough out onto a piece of baking parchment or a lightly floured surface. The dough will be very crumbly and will seem too dry; do not be tempted to add extra liquid. Gently knead the dough a few times until it is well mixed and sticks together.

5. Form the dough into a 15cm (6in) square, about 3cm (1¼in) thick. Dip a knife into some flour and then cut the dough into 4 squares. Cut the squares in half diagonally to form 8 triangles. Arrange on the prepared baking tray.

6. In a small bowl, whisk together the remaining egg with the water. Brush the egg wash on the scones. Bake for 20–25 minutes or until the tops are golden brown. Cool completely on a wire rack before serving, with butter, if you like.

Store it ··

Individually wrap in cling film and store in an airtight container in the freezer for up to 3 months. Defrost at room temperature, or reheat in the oven.

Tip ··

If you use a brand of vegetable fat that contains a lot of water, you may find your scones spreading excessively. Chill the dough for at least 1 hour before baking, to help prevent the spreading.

Makes:
8

Prep time:
15 minutes, plus cooling

Cook time:
25 minutes

These scones will make you feel like royalty enjoying high tea. They have the perfect amount of sweetness with bursts of fresh blueberries and they pair wonderfully with clotted cream and jam. They also freeze very well and are great to have on hand for a quick breakfast.

Afternoon Tea Blueberry Scones

320g (11oz) No. 1 All-Purpose Flour Blend (see p24), plus 1 tbsp, plus extra for dusting

2 tsp xanthan gum

3 tbsp golden granulated sugar, plus extra for topping

1 tbsp baking powder

¾ tsp salt

85g (3oz) white vegetable fat (see tip, below)

150g (5½oz) blueberries (fresh, frozen, or dried)

2 large eggs, lightly beaten

80ml (2½fl oz) canned coconut cream or double cream, plus extra for brushing

1 tsp apple cider vinegar

1. Place the oven shelf in the centre of the oven and preheat it to 200°C (180°C fan/400°F/Gas 6). Line a baking tray with baking parchment. In a large bowl, whisk together the 320g (11¼oz) of No. 1 All-Purpose Flour Blend, the xanthan gum, sugar, baking powder, and salt.

2. Using a pastry cutter or fork, cut in the vegetable fat until pea-sized crumbs are formed. If using fresh or frozen blueberries, toss them in the remaining 1 tablespoon All-Purpose Flour Blend; this will prevent them from sinking to the bottom. Stir in the blueberries.

3. In a separate medium bowl, lightly beat the eggs. Then beat in the coconut cream or double cream, and vinegar.

4. Make a well in the centre of the dry ingredients and pour in the cream mixture. Stir carefully until just combined. The dough will be very crumbly.

5. Turn the dough out onto a piece of baking parchment or a lightly floured surface. The dough will be very crumbly and will seem too dry; do not be tempted to add extra liquid. Gently knead the dough a few times until it is well mixed and sticks together.

6. Form the dough into a 15cm (6in) square about 3cm (1¼in) thick. Dip a knife into some flour and then cut the dough into 4 squares. Cut the squares in half diagonally to form 8 triangles. Arrange on the prepared baking tray.

7. Brush the tops of each scone with coconut cream or double cream and sprinkle with sugar. Bake for 20–25 minutes or until the tops are golden brown. Cool on a wire rack before serving.

Store it
Store in an airtight container for 2–3 days, refrigerate for 5 days, or freeze, individually wrapped, for up to 3 months. Defrost at room temperature, or reheat in the microwave.

Tip
If you use a brand of vegetable fat that contains a lot of water, you may find your scones spreading excessively. Chill the dough for at least 1 hour before baking, to help prevent the spreading.

Makes:
8

Prep time:
25 minutes, plus cooling

Cook time:
25 minutes

Some of the coffee shops where I live start selling maple scones in the autumn. They are pretty incredible. I used to get so excited every year when they started to appear. I have not had a coffee shop scone in a very long time, but this recipe brings me right back to the days of maple scones and lattes on my way to work…

Coffee Shop Maple Scones

320g (11oz) No. 1
  All-Purpose Flour Blend
  (see p24), plus extra
  for dusting

2 tsp xanthan gum

2 tbsp golden granulated
  sugar

1 tbsp baking powder

¾ tsp salt

85g (3oz) white vegetable
  fat (see tip, below)

50g (1¾oz) chopped
  pecans

2 large eggs

80ml (2½fl oz) double
  cream

2 tbsp pure maple syrup

1 tsp apple cider vinegar

For the maple icing

260g (9oz) icing sugar

85g (3oz) pure maple
  syrup

½–1 tbsp whole milk

1. Preheat the oven to 200°C (180°C fan/400°F/Gas 6) and line a baking tray with baking parchment. In a large bowl, whisk together the No. 1 All-Purpose Flour Blend, xanthan gum, sugar, baking powder, and salt.

2. Using a pastry cutter or fork, cut in the vegetable fat until pea-sized crumbs are formed. Stir in the pecans.

3. In a separate medium bowl, lightly beat the eggs. Then beat in the cream, maple syrup, and vinegar.

4. Make a well in the centre of the dry ingredients and pour in the cream mixture. Stir carefully until just combined.

5. Turn the dough out onto a piece of baking parchment or a lightly floured surface. The dough will be very crumbly and will seem too dry; do not be tempted to add extra liquid. Gently knead the dough a few times until it is well mixed and sticks together.

6. Form the dough into a 15cm (6in) square about 3cm (1¼in) thick. Dip a knife into some flour and then cut the dough into 4 squares. Cut the squares in half diagonally to form 8 triangles. Arrange on the prepared baking sheet.

7. Bake for 20–25 minutes or until the tops are golden brown. Cool on a wire rack. Dip the cooled scones in the icing, and let set on the wire rack before serving.

   Maple Icing: In a small bowl, stir together the icing sugar, maple syrup, and ½ tablespoon milk. Add more milk 1 teaspoon at a time until a smooth, thin icing is formed.

Store it
Let the iced scones cool completely. Store in an airtight container for up to 3 days, or individually wrapped in the freezer for up to 3 months. Defrost at room temperature, or reheat in the oven or microwave.

Tip
If you use a brand of vegetable fat that contains a lot of water, you may find your scones spreading excessively. Chill the dough for at least 1 hour before baking, to help prevent the spreading.

Pies & Fruity Desserts

Makes:
2 x 23cm (9in) pie crusts

Prep time:
15 minutes,
plus chilling

Cook time:
None

360g (13oz) No. 1
   All-Purpose Flour Blend
   (see p24), plus extra
   for dusting
1 tsp xanthan gum
2 tbsp golden granulated
   sugar (optional; omit for
   savoury recipes)
170g (6oz) salted butter,
   chilled and chopped
   into 5mm (¼in) pieces
5-7 tbsp ice-cold water
1 egg, for blind-baking
   (optional)

Sometimes the best part of a pie is its buttery, flaky pastry. But let's face it, store-bought pastry cases are anything but buttery, flaky, or tasty, and I'm not even talking here about the gluten-free ones, which are non-existent in the average shop. This is a great multi-purpose pastry for sweet or savoury pies, quiches, or any recipe needing a pastry case.

Buttery Pastry

1. Put the No. 1 All-Purpose Flour Blend in a food processor with the xanthan gum and sugar (if using). Pulse until combined. Add the butter and pulse until the mixture resembles a coarse meal.

2. Add the ice-cold water 1 tablespoon at a time, pulsing to combine after each addition. The pastry should hold together when squeezed, but not be too sticky.

3. Divide and shape the pastry into 2 even discs. Wrap each half separately in cling film and refrigerate for at least 2 hours, or up to 2 days. (The pastry can be frozen at this point, too, and used within 3 months.)

4. Before baking, remove the discs from the refrigerator and let sit at room temperature for 5–10 minutes. Place the discs between 2 sheets of baking parchment, silicone baking mats, or 2 sheets of floured cling film. Roll out into a 30cm (12in) circle, 1.5–3mm (¹⁄₁₆–¹⁄₈in) thick. If it begins to stick to the surface, lightly flour the work surface and the top of the pastry.

5. Either blind-bake the pastry case (see below) or proceed using the raw rolled-out pastry, as directed by the recipe.

    Blind-Bake: Mould a pastry circle into a pie dish and freeze for 30 minutes. (Leave the other pastry circle in the refrigerator, if using.) Position the oven shelf in the lower one-third of the oven. Place a baking tray on the rack and preheat the oven to 200°C (180°C fan/400°F/Gas 6). In a small bowl, whisk together 1 egg and 1 tablespoon water. Brush the edge of the pastry case with the egg wash. Line the case with baking parchment and baking beans, and bake for 20 minutes on the hot baking tray. Remove the baking parchment and baking beans, and bake for 5 minutes more.

Tip ....

This recipe makes enough pastry for two pie crusts. If you only need one, or are making extra pastry, wrap the rest in cling film and store in the freezer. That way you have it available any time you feel like making a pie.

Makes:
1 x 23cm (9in) pie

Prep time:
30 minutes

Cook time:
1 hour

1 raw Buttery Pastry disc
(see left)
vanilla ice cream, to serve

For the topping

240g (8½oz) No. 1
All-Purpose Flour Blend
(see p24)
1 tsp xanthan gum
130g (4½oz) light brown
sugar
½ tsp ground cinnamon
170g (6oz) salted butter,
chilled and chopped
into small pieces

For the filling

200g (7oz) golden
granulated sugar
40g (1½oz) No. 1
All-Purpose Flour Blend
(see p24)
½ tsp xanthan gum
pinch of ground nutmeg
2 tsp ground cinnamon
dash of salt
6-8 peeled, cored,
and sliced tart apples,
such as Granny Smith,
1.4-1.75kg (3-4lb)
in total

My mum has always made the most amazing apple pie with a crumble topping. It was a staple of our Thanksgiving dinners, and I would always save room for it. I think my favourite part was having a slice for breakfast the next morning! This recipe is the gluten-free version of my mum's famous pie.

Mum's Apple Pie

1. Roll out the pastry and use it to line a 23cm (9in) deep pie dish. Freeze for 30 minutes.

2. Preheat the oven to 220°C (200°C fan/425°F/Gas 7). Prepare the topping. In a small bowl, stir together the No. 1 All-Purpose Flour Blend, xanthan gum, brown sugar, and cinnamon until combined. Using a fork or your hands, cut in the cold butter until it is well dispersed and pea-sized crumbs are formed. Set aside.

3. Prepare the filling. In a large bowl, stir together the sugar, No. 1 All-Purpose Flour Blend, xanthan gum, nutmeg, cinnamon, and salt. Stir in the apples until well coated.

4. Pour the apples into the prepared pastry case, mounding them up high. Evenly spoon the crumble topping over the apples, spreading it until they are all covered, and press down lightly.

5. Bake for 50–60 minutes or until golden brown and the apples are soft when pierced with a fork. Cover the pie with foil for the last 20–25 minutes if the topping starts to get too brown.

6. Cool on a wire rack. Serve warm or at room temperature with vanilla ice cream.

Store it ....
Cover with cling film, or transfer to an airtight container, and refrigerate for up to 3 days.

Makes:
1 x 23cm (9in) pie

Prep time:
20 minutes, plus chilling

Cook time:
1 hour 10 minutes

1 raw Buttery Pastry disc
(see p138)

200g (7oz) golden
granulated sugar

3 tbsp light brown sugar

½ tsp salt

340g (12oz) golden syrup

75g (2½oz) salted butter,
melted and cooled

1 tsp vanilla extract

3 large eggs

125g (4½oz) chopped
pecans

Pecan is usually my pie of choice, and this version satisfies me. It's incredibly sweet, chewy, and delicious, and pairs perfectly with vanilla ice cream. When I was selling my baked goods to local shops, this pie was a huge hit and so easy to make.

Pecan Pie

1. Roll out the pastry and use it to line a 23cm (9in) deep pie dish. Freeze for 30 minutes. Meanwhile, preheat the oven to 180°C (160°C fan/350°F/Gas 4).

2. In a medium bowl, whisk together the granulated sugar, brown sugar, salt, golden syrup, melted butter, vanilla, and eggs until well combined.

3. Remove the pastry case from the freezer and spread the chopped pecans in it. Pour the sugar mixture over the nuts.

4. Lightly cover with foil without letting the foil touch the pie filling and bake for 40 minutes. Remove the foil and bake for 20–30 minutes more, or until the filling is set. Let cool completely before cutting. Serve at room temperature.

Store it ⋯⋯⋯⋯⋯⋯⋯⋯⋯⋯⋯⋯⋯⋯⋯⋯⋯⋯⋯⋯⋯⋯⋯⋯⋯⋯⋯⋯⋯

Cover with cling film, or transfer to an airtight container, and refrigerate for up to 5 days.

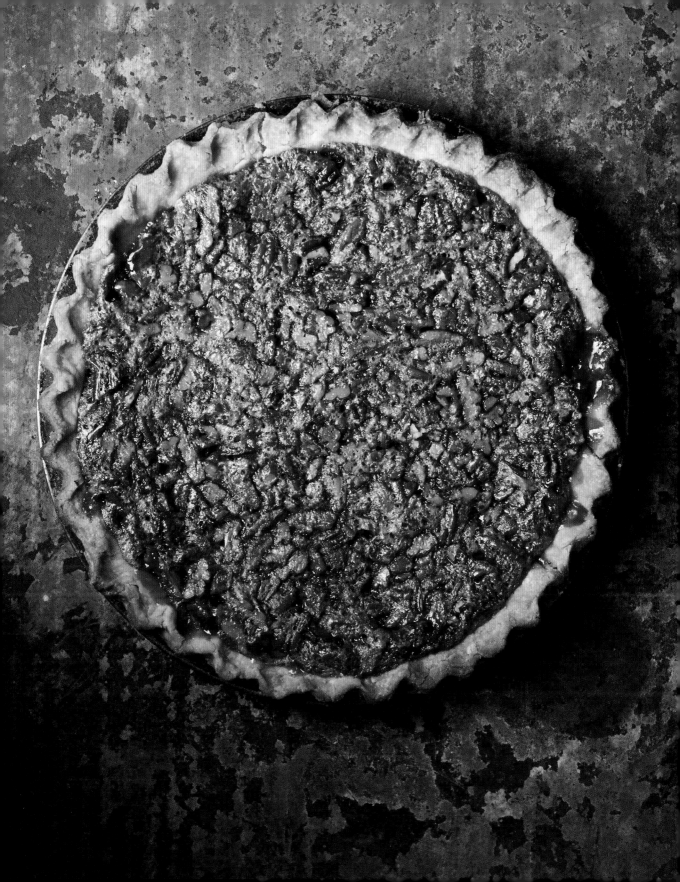

Makes:
1 x 23cm (9in) pie

Prep time:
10 minutes,
plus cooling

Cook time:
1 hour 5 minutes

1 raw Buttery Pastry disc
(see p138)
150g (5½oz) golden
granulated sugar
½ tsp salt
1 tsp ground cinnamon
¼ tsp ground ginger
¼ tsp ground nutmeg
⅛ tsp ground cloves
2 large eggs
400g can 100 per cent
pure pumpkin
350ml can evaporated
milk

American Thanksgiving is not complete unless you smell pumpkin pie baking in the oven. This is a great pie to make for your gluten-eating friends because, with its naturally gluten-free filling and flaky pastry, it's just as good as any other version out there.

Pumpkin Pie

1. Preheat the oven to 220°C (200°C fan/425°F/Gas 7). Roll out the pastry and use it to line a 23cm (9in) deep pie dish.

2. In a small bowl, mix together the sugar, salt, cinnamon, ginger, nutmeg, and cloves.

3. In a stand mixer fitted with the paddle attachment, or in a large bowl, beat the eggs on high speed. Stir in the pumpkin and the sugar mixture. Gradually whisk in the evaporated milk.

4. Pour the filling into the prepared pastry case. Bake for 15 minutes and then reduce the oven temperature to 180°C (160°C fan/350°F/Gas 4). Continue to bake for another 40–50 minutes or until a knife inserted near the centre comes out clean. If the edges of the pastry start to get too dark, cover them with foil.

5. Cool on a wire rack for 2 hours and then store in the refrigerator. Serve cold or at room temperature.

Store it ···

Cover with cling film, or transfer to an airtight container, and refrigerate for up to 5 days.

Makes:
1 x 23cm (9in) pie

Prep time:
20 minutes, plus chilling

Cook time:
10 minutes

1.8kg (4lb) fresh
strawberries, hulled
150g (5½oz) golden
granulated sugar
1½ tbsp cornflour
1½ tsp powdered gelatine
pinch of salt
1 tbsp lemon juice
1 blind-baked Buttery
Pastry case (see p138)

**For the whipped cream
topping**
240ml (8fl oz) double
cream
4 tbsp icing sugar
1 tsp vanilla extract
1 tsp powdered gelatine
1 tbsp water

Growing up in California, we would often buy strawberry pies for special occasions. It was always my favourite (and my brother's). Now, when strawberry season rolls around, I make my own version. This is best served within 6 hours of making.

Fresh Strawberry Pie

1. Chop 190g (6¾oz) of the strawberries, leaving the rest whole. In a food processor or blender, process the chopped strawberries into a smooth purée. (You should have about 175g/6oz purée.)

2. In a medium saucepan over a medium-high heat, whisk together the strawberry purée, sugar, cornflour, gelatine, and salt until well combined. Continue cooking and stirring constantly until the mixture comes to a full boil. Boil for 2 minutes, constantly stirring and scraping the bottom and sides of the pan to prevent burning. After boiling for 2 minutes, pour the mixture into a large bowl.

3. Whisk in the lemon juice. Let the glaze cool to room temperature.

4. Cut any extra-large strawberries in half. Gently fold all the remaining strawberries into the cooled glaze until they are well coated.

5. Spoon the strawberries into the cooled pastry case and pile into a large mound. Refrigerate for 2 hours. Using a pastry bag with a large icing tip, pipe the whipped cream topping onto the chilled pie, or just dollop it onto each slice before serving.

Whipped Cream Topping:

1. In the bowl of a stand mixer, or in a large metal bowl, stir together the cream, icing sugar, and vanilla. Refrigerate the bowl along with the whisk attachment for 5 minutes.

2. While the mixture is chilling, in a small microwave-safe bowl, combine the gelatine with the measured water. When the gelatine has completely absorbed the water, microwave the mixture for 15 seconds to liquefy. Stir and let sit until it reaches room temperature.

3. Remove the bowl from the refrigerator. Using the chilled whisk attachment, beat the cream mixture on medium-high until soft peaks form. Slowly drizzle in the liquid gelatine mixture. (If the gelatine has hardened up, microwave for a few seconds until liquid again, but be sure it cools a bit before adding.) Beat until stiff peaks form. Refrigerate until ready to use.

Store it ··

This pie is best eaten on the day it's made. To store, cover with cling film and refrigerate for 1–2 days.

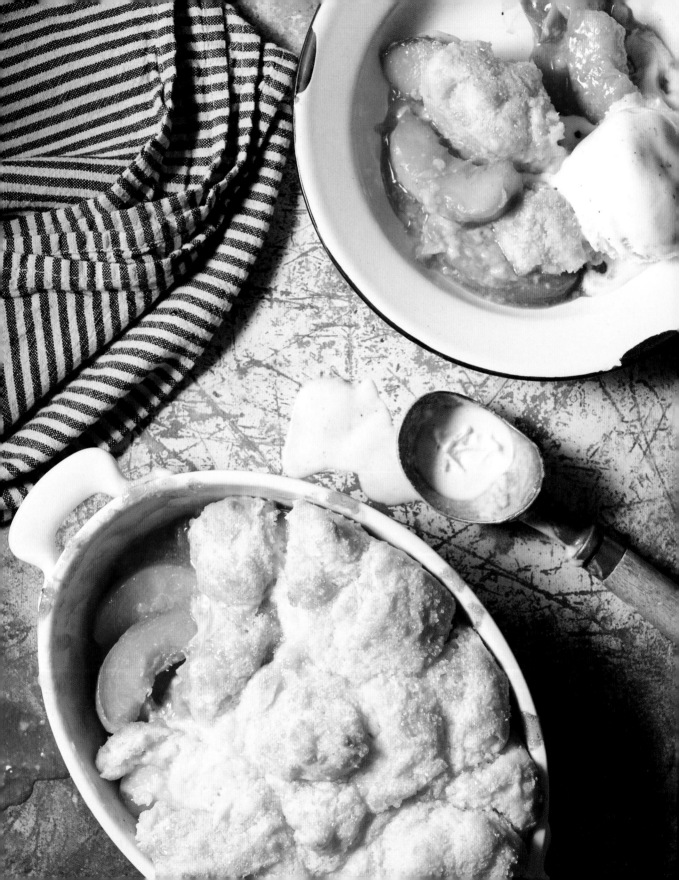

Serves:
6

Prep time:
30 minutes

Cook time:
45 minutes

vanilla ice cream, to serve

For the filling

8–10 small or 5–6 large
  peaches, pitted and
  sliced, 875g–1kg
  (2–2¼lb) in total
1 tsp lemon juice
60g (2oz) golden
  granulated sugar
1 tbsp cornflour
¼ tsp ground cinnamon
60ml (2fl oz) water

For the topping

200g (7oz) No. 1
  All-Purpose Flour Blend
  (see p24)
½ tsp xanthan gum
60g (2oz) golden
  granulated sugar
½ tsp salt
1 tbsp baking powder
60g (2oz) salted butter,
  melted and cooled
2 tsp vanilla extract
1 tsp apple cider vinegar
180ml (6fl oz) whole milk
demerara sugar, for
  sprinkling

During peach season, we make this cobbler over and over again in my house. My favourite way to eat it is slightly warm with a scoop of vanilla ice cream. This gluten-free version tastes just as good for breakfast the next morning.

Peach Cobbler

1. Preheat the oven to 190°C (170°C fan/375°F/Gas 5) and prepare the peach filling. In a medium saucepan, stir together the peaches, lemon juice, sugar, cornflour, cinnamon, and measured water over a medium-high heat. Bring to the boil and cook until the peaches start to soften and the liquid is slightly thick, 8–10 minutes. Pour into a 2 litre (3½ pint) baking dish.

2. Prepare the topping. In a medium bowl, whisk together the No. 1 All-Purpose Flour Blend, xanthan gum, sugar, salt, and baking powder.

3. In a separate medium bowl, whisk together the melted butter, vanilla, vinegar, and milk until well combined.

4. Pour the wet ingredients into the flour mixture and stir until well combined. Let sit for 2–3 minutes to slightly thicken up. Arrange the topping over the peach mixture. Sprinkle with demerara sugar.

5. Bake for 30–35 minutes or until the peaches are very soft, the topping is golden brown, and a toothpick inserted into the topping comes out clean. Serve warm or at room temperature with a scoop of vanilla ice cream.

Store it ···
Store in an airtight container in the refrigerator for up to 5 days. Eat leftovers cold, at room temperature, or slightly warmed up in the microwave or oven.

Tip ···
If it's not peach season, you can substitute frozen sliced peaches for the fresh peaches. Defrost the peaches before using.

Makes:
33 x 23cm (13 x 9in) cheesecake

Prep time:
30 minutes, plus chilling

Cook time:
15 minutes

2 x 595g cans cherry pie filling (gluten-free; available online)

For the crust
225g (8oz) salted butter, softened
320g (11oz) No. 1 All-Purpose Flour Blend (see p24)
85g (3oz) light brown sugar
1 tsp xanthan gum
100g (3½oz) pecans or walnuts, finely chopped

For the filling
225g (8oz) cream cheese, at room temperature
130g (4¾oz) icing sugar
1 tsp vanilla extract
340g (12oz) sweetened squirty cream, or sweetened whipped cream

Growing up, we served this cheesecake at most parties, and it was always a firm favourite. Cheesecakes can sometimes be tricky to make, but with this foolproof recipe, it'll only seem like you spent hours preparing it. The sweet, creamy cheese layer against the tart cherries is the perfect combination.

Cherry Cheesecake

1. Preheat the oven to 180°C (160°C fan/350°F/Gas 4). Make the crust. Put the butter in a large bowl with the No. 1 All-Purpose Flour Blend, brown sugar, xanthan gum, and nuts. Using your hands, mix the ingredients together until well combined.

2. Pour the crust mixture into a 33 x 23cm (13 x 9in) baking dish, and press evenly into the dish. Bake for 15 minutes. Let cool completely.

3. Prepare the filling. Put the cream cheese in a stand mixer fitted with the paddle attachment, or in a large bowl, and add the icing sugar, vanilla, and cream. Beat on medium-high speed until well combined and smooth.

4. When the crust has cooled, spread the filling evenly over. Spread the cherry pie filling evenly over the top. Chill in the refrigerator for 2 hours. Cut into squares and serve.

Store it ···
Cover with cling film and refrigerate for up to 5 days.

Tip ···
Substitute strawberry or blueberry gluten-free pie filling for the cherry pie filling, if desired.

Serves:
9–12

Prep time:
20 minutes

Cook time:
40 minutes

5 medium Granny Smith
   apples, peeled, cored,
   and chopped (roughly
   1.25cm/½in pieces)

190g (6¾oz) light brown
   sugar

120g (4½oz) No. 1
   All-Purpose Flour Blend
   (see p24)

75g (2½oz) rolled oats
   (certified gluten-free)

1 tsp ground cinnamon

1 tsp xanthan gum

½ tsp ground nutmeg

115g (4oz) salted butter,
   cut into cubes and
   slightly softened

vanilla ice cream or
   whipped cream
   (optional), to serve

In my opinion, the topping is always the best part of any type of crisp. When creating this recipe, I made sure that every bite of apple had an ample amount of crispy, sweet topping. Because the ingredients are simple staples, it's a great last-minute dessert.

Apple Crisp

1. Preheat the oven to 190°C (170°C fan/375°F/Gas 5). Spread the apples in a 20 or 23cm (8 or 9in) square oven dish.

2. In a medium bowl, stir together the brown sugar, No. 1 All-Purpose Flour Blend, oats, cinnamon, xanthan gum, and nutmeg until well combined.

3. Using a pastry cutter or your hands, cut in the butter until pea-sized crumbs are formed.

4. Evenly sprinkle the topping over the apples. Bake for 35–40 minutes or until the topping is golden brown and the apples are soft when pierced with a fork.

5. Let cool for at least 10 minutes before serving. Serve warm by itself, or topped with vanilla ice cream or whipped cream.

Store it

Cover with cling film and refrigerate for up to 3 days. Enjoy chilled, at room temperature, or slightly reheated in the oven or microwave (my favourite).

Makes:
1 x 23cm (9in) tart

Prep time:
30 minutes, plus cooling and chilling

Cook time:
30 minutes

1 raw Buttery Pastry disc (see p138)

4 pears

1 tsp lemon juice

225g (8oz) cream cheese, softened

50g (1¾oz) golden granulated sugar

1 large egg

1 tsp vanilla extract

For the glaze

85g (3oz) apricot jam

½ tsp vanilla extract

½ tsp lemon juice

2 tbsp water

This dessert is sure to impress your friends. It's so easy to make and yet so beautiful with the wheel of pears on top. The sweetness of the glaze and pears is perfect with the cream cheese filling. A scoop of vanilla ice cream is amazing to top it off.

Pear Tart

1. Roll out the pastry and use it to line a 23cm (9in) deep pie dish. Freeze for 30 minutes. Meanwhile, preheat the oven to 190°C (170°C fan/375°F/Gas 5).

2. Once the pastry case is frozen, line it with a sheet of baking parchment and fill with baking beans. Bake for 10 minutes.

3. While the crust is baking, prepare the pears and filling. Peel and thinly slice the pears (about 5mm/¼in thick) and toss with the lemon juice. Set aside.

4. After baking the crust, increase the oven temperature to 220°C (200°C fan/425°F/Gas 7). In a stand mixer fitted with the paddle attachment, or in a medium bowl, beat the cream cheese and sugar on high speed until smooth. Beat in the egg and vanilla until combined.

5. Spread the filling into the par-baked crust. Arrange the pears on top of the filling in a circular pattern.

6. Bake the tart for 10 minutes. Reduce the heat to 180°C (160°C fan/350°F/Gas 4) and continue baking for 15–20 minutes, or until the filling is set.

7. While the tart is baking, prepare the glaze. In a small saucepan, cook the apricot jam, vanilla, lemon juice, and measured water over a medium heat for 6–8 minutes or until melted and smooth. Strain out the solids, if desired. Preheat the grill on its highest setting.

8. Brush the glaze onto the pears. Grill the tart for 1–2 minutes or until shiny, being careful not to let it burn.

9. Cool the tart on a wire rack for 1 hour. Transfer to the refrigerator and chill for at least 2 hours before serving. Serve cold.

Store it ....
Store in an airtight container in the refrigerator for up to 5 days.

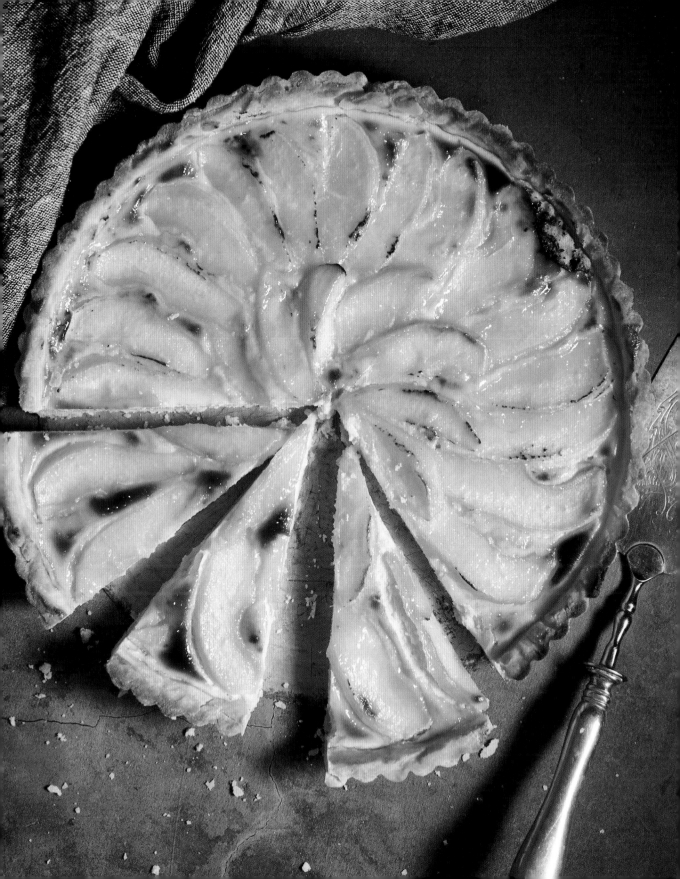

Cakes & Cupcakes

Makes:
32

Prep time:
30 minutes, plus cooling

Cook time:
25 minutes

Sending your gluten-free child to a party is always a bit tricky, especially when it's time for cake. I never wanted my children to miss out, so I made a chocolate cupcake that was equally good (if not better) than the gluten-filled cupcakes being served. Mission accomplished! You can also use this recipe to make a cake.

Chocolate Cupcakes

400g (14oz) golden granulated sugar

225g (8oz) salted butter, softened

3 large eggs, at room temperature

400g (14oz) No. 1 All-Purpose Flour Blend (see p24)

½ tsp salt

1½ tsp baking powder

½ tsp bicarbonate of soda

120g (4½oz) cocoa powder

2 tsp xanthan gum

120ml (4fl oz) brewed coffee, hot or cold

240ml (8fl oz) whole milk

2 tsp vanilla extract

2 tsp apple cider vinegar

For the chocolate buttercream frosting

340g (12oz) salted butter, softened

120g (4½oz) cocoa powder

650–780g (1lb 7oz–1lb 12oz) icing sugar, plus extra if needed

6–8 tbsp double cream

1 tsp vanilla extract

1. Preheat the oven to 180°C (160°C fan/350°F/Gas 4) and line the muffin tins with paper cases. In a stand mixer fitted with the paddle attachment, or in a large bowl, cream the sugar and butter on medium-high speed until light and fluffy, 3–5 minutes.

2. Beat in the eggs one at a time until incorporated. In a separate medium bowl, sift together the No. 1 All-Purpose Flour Blend, salt, baking powder, bicarbonate of soda, cocoa powder, and xanthan gum.

3. Slowly beat the dry ingredients into the butter mixture on low speed until combined. While on low speed, slowly add the coffee, milk, vanilla, and vinegar, and beat until well combined.

4. Using an ice-cream scoop, fill each muffin case about two-thirds full. Bake for 20–25 minutes or until the cupcakes spring back when touched and a toothpick inserted into the centres comes out clean.

5. Cool in the tins for 3 minutes and then transfer to a wire rack to cool completely. Once completely cooled, frost the cupcakes (see tip, right).

Chocolate Buttercream Frosting: In a stand mixer fitted with the paddle attachment, or in a large bowl, beat the butter for 1 minute on high speed. On low speed, slowly add the cocoa powder and beat until well combined. Add half the icing sugar. Increase the speed to high and beat for 2 minutes. Then add 6 tablespoons of the cream, the vanilla, and the remaining icing sugar. Beat on low speed to incorporate, and then increase the speed to high and beat for 3–5 minutes. Beat in more sugar or cream as needed to reach the desired consistency.

Chocolate Cake: Grease and lightly flour only the bases of two 23cm (9in) round cake tins. Portion equal amounts of batter into each cake tin, gently tapping them on the work surface to evenly spread. Bake for 40–45 minutes or until a toothpick inserted into the centres comes out clean. Let cool in the tins on a wire rack for 10 minutes. Remove from the tins and cool completely on a wire rack. Frost once completely cooled.

Store it

Store the frosted cupcakes in an airtight container in the refrigerator for up to 1 day, or in the freezer for up to 3 months. Defrost at room temperature.

Makes:
24

Prep time:
30 minutes, plus cooling

Cook time:
25 minutes

If you're either chocolate or vanilla, then I'm definitely vanilla. A fluffy white cake with buttercream frosting has always been my favourite. This recipe took many attempts to create but was so worth the effort. Whenever I serve these cupcakes to family and friends, they're shocked they're gluten-free because they're so moist and light.

Vanilla Cupcakes

400g (14oz) golden granulated sugar

225g (8oz) salted butter, at room temperature

4 large eggs, separated

2 tsp vanilla extract

480g (1lb 1oz) No. 2 All-Purpose Flour Blend (see p24)

1½ tsp xanthan gum

1 tbsp baking powder

2 tsp apple cider vinegar

240ml (8fl oz) whole milk

For the buttercream frosting

340g (12oz) salted butter, softened

780–910g (1lb 12oz–2lb) icing sugar

6–8 tbsp double cream

1½ tsp vanilla extract

1. Preheat the oven to 180°C (160°C fan/350°F/Gas 4) and line the muffin tins with paper cases. In a stand mixer fitted with the paddle attachment, or in a large bowl, cream the sugar and butter on medium-high speed until light and fluffy, 3–5 minutes.

2. Beat in the egg yolks one at a time until incorporated, then beat in the vanilla. In a separate bowl, combine the No. 2 All-Purpose Flour Blend, xanthan gum, and baking powder. Add to the butter mixture and mix well on low speed.

3. In a separate small bowl, beat the egg whites on high speed until stiff peaks form.

4. On low speed, mix the vinegar and milk into the cake batter. Gently fold the egg whites into the batter.

5. Using an ice-cream scoop, fill each muffin case about two-thirds full. Bake for 20–25 minutes or until the cupcakes spring back when touched and a toothpick inserted into the centres comes out clean.

6. Cool in the tins for 5 minutes and then transfer to a wire rack to cool completely. Once completely cooled, frost the cupcakes.

   Buttercream Frosting: In a stand mixer fitted with the paddle attachment, or in a large bowl, beat the butter for 1 minute on high speed. On low speed, slowly add 390g (14oz) of the icing sugar. Increase the speed to high and beat for 2 minutes. Then add 6 tablespoons of the cream, the vanilla, and 390g (14oz) more icing sugar. Beat on low speed to incorporate, and then increase the speed to high and beat for 3–5 minutes. Beat in more sugar or cream as needed to reach the desired consistency.

Store it

Store the frosted cupcakes in an airtight container in the refrigerator for up to 2 days, or in the freezer for up to 3 months. Defrost at room temperature.

Tips

To frost the cupcakes, use a piping bag and a large icing tip for the prettiest result! My favourite icing tip is a Wilton 1M open star icing tip.

I like to keep a few of these in the freezer at all times so I'm always prepared for when my kids are invited to a party. I can send them with their own cupcake in a small airtight container, and then they are not left out at cake time.

Makes:
24

Prep time:
30 minutes, plus cooling

Cook time:
25 minutes

400g (14oz) golden granulated sugar

225g (8oz) salted butter, softened

4 large eggs, separated

3 tsp vanilla extract

480g (1lb 1oz) No. 2 All-Purpose Flour Blend (see p24)

1½ tsp xanthan gum

3 tsp baking powder

240ml (8fl oz) whole milk

1 tsp apple cider vinegar

For the filling

450g (1lb) strawberries, roughly chopped

240ml (8fl oz) double cream

45g (1½oz) icing sugar, plus extra for dusting

These cupcakes are a variation of a strawberry shortcake, conveniently transformed into a hand-held cake. The whipped cream frosting is also more delicate than buttercream frosting, creating a lighter dessert than my vanilla cupcake.

Strawberry Shortcake Cupcakes

1. Preheat the oven to 180°C (160°C fan/350°F/Gas 4) and line the muffin tins with paper cases. In a stand mixer fitted with the paddle attachment, or in a large bowl, cream the sugar and butter on medium-high speed until light and fluffy, 3–5 minutes.

2. Beat in the egg yolks and vanilla until combined. In a medium bowl, whisk together the No. 2 All-Purpose Flour Blend, xanthan gum, and baking powder. Add the dry mixture to the wet mixture and mix well on low speed. Stir in the milk and vinegar.

3. In a separate medium bowl, beat the egg whites on high speed until soft peaks form. Gently fold the egg whites into the batter.

4. Using an ice-cream scoop, fill each muffin case about two-thirds full. Bake for 20–25 minutes or until the cupcakes spring back when touched and a toothpick inserted into the centres comes out clean. Cool in the tins for 5 minutes, and then transfer to a wire rack to cool completely.

5. While the cupcakes are cooling, make the filling. In a medium bowl, use a fork or potato masher to mash the chopped strawberries. In a stand mixer fitted with the whisk attachment, or in a separate medium bowl, beat the cream and icing sugar until stiff peaks form. Drain the strawberries and then fold the mashed strawberries into the whipped cream.

6. Assemble the cupcakes. Carefully remove the paper case from each cupcake and cut the domed top off each. Spoon about 2 tablespoons of the strawberry cream mixture on top of each cupcake base. Place the cupcake tops back on each cupcake. Dust the tops with icing sugar. Serve immediately.

Store it
Cover the assembled cupcakes with cling film and refrigerate for up to 2 days. I do not recommend freezing these cupcakes because of the delicate filling.

Tip
You can make both the cupcakes and the filling up to 1 day in advance and store in separate airtight containers in the refrigerator. Assemble the cupcakes just before serving.

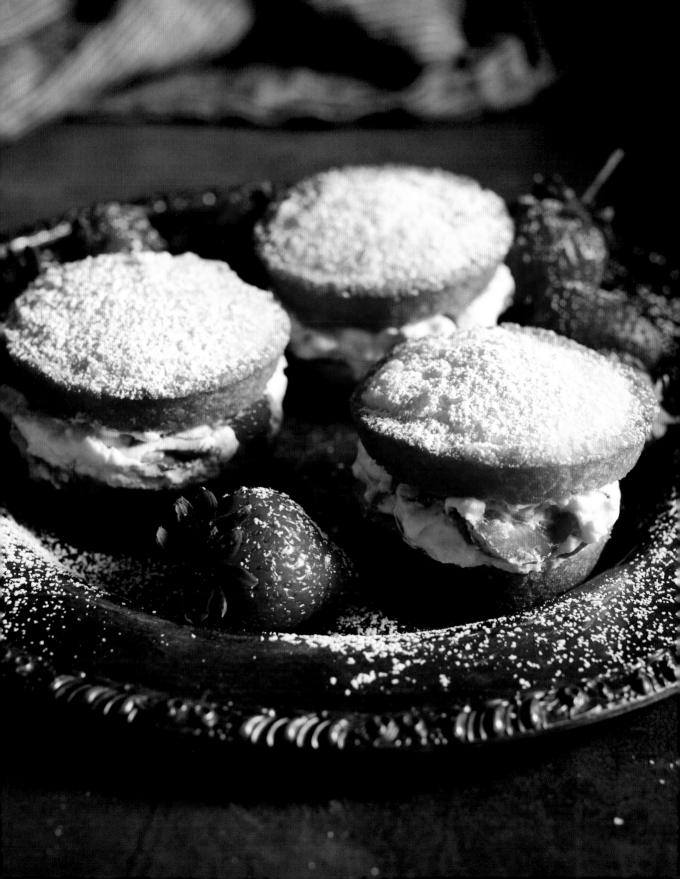

Looking to move on from baking plain vanilla cupcakes? These would be an amazing upgrade. The raspberry buttercream frosting makes them so pretty and complements the lemon flavour perfectly.

Lemon Cupcakes
with Raspberry Buttercream

400g (14oz) golden
 granulated sugar

225g (8oz) salted butter,
 softened

4 large eggs, separated

finely grated zest of
 1 unwaxed lemon

2 tbsp lemon juice

480g (1lb 1oz) No. 2
 All-Purpose Flour Blend
 (see p24)

1½ tsp xanthan gum

1 tbsp baking powder

2 tsp apple cider vinegar

240ml (8fl oz) whole milk

**For the raspberry
buttercream frosting**

175g (6oz) raspberries

340g (12oz) salted butter,
 softened

780–910g (1lb 12oz–2lb)
 icing sugar

6-8 tbsp double cream

1½ tsp vanilla extract

1. Preheat the oven to 180°C (160°C fan/350°F/Gas 4) and line the muffin tins with paper cases. In a stand mixer fitted with the paddle attachment, or in a large bowl, cream the sugar and butter on medium-high speed until light and fluffy, 3–5 minutes. Beat in the egg yolks, lemon zest, and lemon juice on medium-high speed until well combined.

2. In a separate medium bowl, whisk together the No. 2 All-Purpose Flour Blend, xanthan gum, and baking powder. Add the dry mixture to the wet mixture and mix well on low speed.

3. In another separate medium bowl, beat the egg whites until stiff peaks form.

4. On low speed, mix the vinegar and milk into the cake batter. Gently fold the egg whites into the batter.

5. Using an ice-cream scoop, fill each muffin case about two-thirds full. Bake for 20–25 minutes or until the cupcakes spring back when touched and a toothpick inserted into the centres comes out clean.

6. Cool in the tins for 5 minutes and then transfer to a wire rack to cool completely. Once completely cooled, frost the cupcakes.

Raspberry Buttercream Frosting: In a blender or food processor, purée the raspberries and then pour through a fine-meshed sieve, discarding the solids. In a stand mixer fitted with the paddle attachment, or in a large bowl, beat the butter for 1 minute on high speed. On low speed, slowly add 390g (14oz) of the icing sugar. Increase the speed to high and beat for 2 minutes. Add the raspberry purée, 6 tablespoons of the cream, the vanilla, and 390g (14oz) more of the icing sugar. Beat on low speed to incorporate, and then increase the speed to high and beat for 3–5 minutes. Beat in more sugar or cream as needed to reach the desired consistency.

Store it ⋯⋯⋯⋯⋯⋯⋯⋯⋯⋯⋯⋯⋯⋯⋯⋯⋯⋯⋯⋯⋯⋯⋯⋯⋯⋯⋯⋯

Store the frosted cupcakes in an airtight container in the refrigerator for up to 1 day, or in the freezer for up to 3 months. Defrost at room temperature.

Tip ⋯⋯⋯⋯⋯⋯⋯⋯⋯⋯⋯⋯⋯⋯⋯⋯⋯⋯⋯⋯⋯⋯⋯⋯⋯⋯⋯⋯⋯⋯⋯⋯

To frost the cupcakes, use a piping bag and a large icing tip for the prettiest result. My favourite icing tip is a Wilton 1M open star icing tip.

Makes:
24

Prep time:
50 minutes, plus cooling

Cook time:
25 minutes

400g (14oz) golden granulated sugar

115g (4oz) salted butter, softened

3 large eggs, at room temperature

400g (14oz) No. 1 All-Purpose Flour Blend (see p24)

½ tsp salt

1½ tsp baking powder

½ tsp bicarbonate of soda

120g (4½oz) cocoa powder

2 tsp xanthan gum

120ml (4fl oz) brewed coffee, hot or cold

240ml (8fl oz) whole milk

2 tsp vanilla extract

2 tsp apple cider vinegar

595g can cherry pie filling (gluten-free; available online)

milk or dark chocolate bar, finely grated, for decorating

24 maraschino cherries, or fresh cherries with stems

For the whipped cream frosting

1½ tsp powdered gelatine

2 tbsp water

360ml (12fl oz) double cream

45g (1½oz) icing sugar

1 tsp vanilla extract

With brewed coffee and cherry pie filling, I think of these cupcakes as the grown-up version of a standard chocolate cupcake. They're so pretty with chocolate shavings and a cherry on top, and the whipped cream frosting is light and yummy.

Black Forest Cupcakes

1. Preheat the oven to 180°C (160°C fan/350°F/Gas 4) and line the muffin tins with paper cases. In a stand mixer fitted with the paddle attachment, or in a large bowl, cream the sugar and butter on medium-high speed until light and fluffy, 3–5 minutes.

2. Beat in the eggs one at a time until incorporated. In a separate medium bowl, whisk together the No. 1 All-Purpose Flour Blend, salt, baking powder, bicarbonate of soda, cocoa powder, and xanthan gum. On low speed, beat the dry ingredients into the wet mixture until combined.

3. On low speed, slowly add the coffee, milk, vanilla, and vinegar. Increase the speed to medium and beat until well combined, scraping down the sides of the bowl as needed. Let the batter rest for 5 minutes.

4. Using a large ice-cream scoop, fill each muffin case about two-thirds full. Bake for 20–25 minutes or until the cupcakes spring back when touched and a toothpick inserted into the centres comes out clean.

5. Cool in the tins for 5 minutes and then transfer to a wire rack to cool completely. Once completely cooled, cut out a small cone-shaped hole in the middle of each cupcake, discarding the removed portion. Fill each hole with cherry pie filling. Using an icing bag with a large icing tip, pipe on the whipped cream frosting (see tip, left). Top with chocolate shavings and a maraschino or fresh cherry. Refrigerate until ready to serve.

Whipped Cream Frosting: In a small microwave-safe bowl, combine the gelatine with the measured water. When the gelatine has completely absorbed the water, microwave the mixture for 15 seconds to liquefy. Stir and let sit until it reaches room temperature. In the bowl of a stand mixer fitted with the whisk attachment, or in a large bowl, beat the cream, icing sugar, and vanilla on medium-high speed. As it starts to thicken, slowly drizzle in the liquid gelatine mixture. (If the gelatine has hardened up, microwave for a few seconds until liquid again, but be sure it cools a bit before adding.) Beat until stiff peaks form. Refrigerate until ready to use.

Store it

Store in an airtight container in the refrigerator for up to 2 days. I do not recommend freezing these cupcakes because of the delicate frosting.

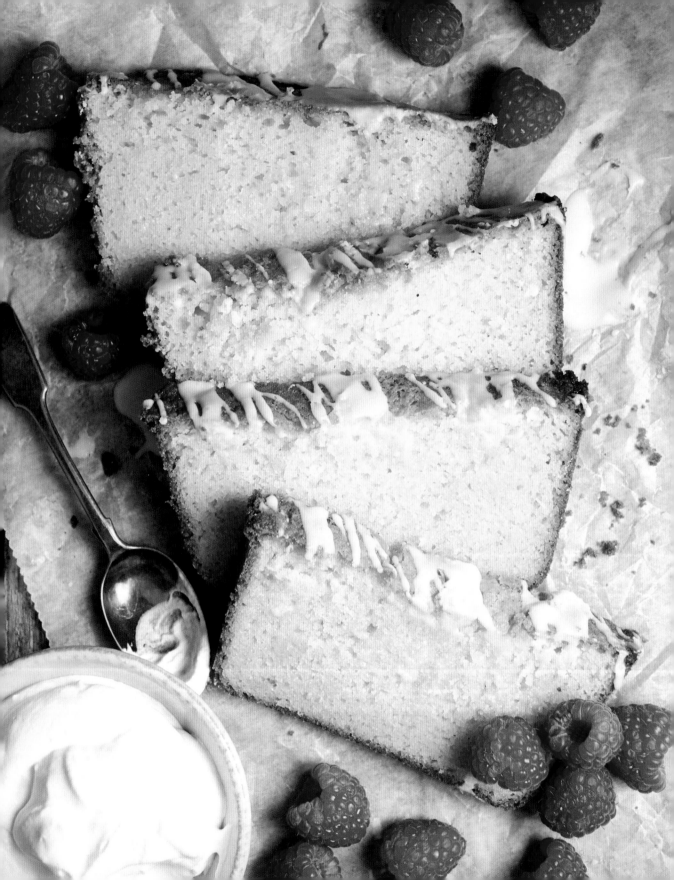

Makes:
1 x 23cm (9in) loaf

Prep time:
15 minutes, plus cooling

Cook time:
55 minutes

175g (6oz) salted butter,
    softened, plus extra
    for greasing
300g (10oz) golden
    granulated sugar
3 large eggs
2 tbsp lemon juice
finely grated zest of
    1 unwaxed lemon
1 tsp vanilla extract
320g (11oz) No. 1
    All-Purpose Flour Blend
    (see p24)
1 tsp baking powder
½ tsp bicarbonate of soda
½ tsp salt
2 tsp xanthan gum
120ml (4fl oz) sour cream
fresh raspberries, or sliced
    strawberries, whipped
    cream, and icing sugar
    (optional), to serve

For the glaze
130g (4¾oz) icing sugar
1 tbsp lemon juice
2 tsp light vegetable oil
    (such as avocado oil)
2 tsp water

This pound cake is amazing with fresh strawberries or raspberries piled on top with icing sugar or whipped cream, and one of my all-time favourite desserts. I created this loaf cake to add to the selection of flavoured loaves I was selling, and it became very popular, especially during the strawberry season.

Lemon Pound Cake

1. Place the oven shelf in the lower third of the oven and preheat the oven to 180°C (160°C fan/350°F/Gas 4). Lightly grease only the base of a 23 x 12.5cm (9 x 5in) loaf tin.

2. In a stand mixer fitted with the paddle attachment, or in a large bowl, cream the butter and sugar, starting on low speed and gradually increasing to high speed, until light and fluffy, 3–5 minutes.

3. Beat in the eggs one at a time until incorporated. Beat in the lemon juice, lemon zest, and vanilla until fully incorporated.

4. In a separate medium bowl, whisk together the No. 1 All-Purpose Flour Blend, baking powder, bicarbonate of soda, salt, and xanthan gum.

5. On low speed, alternate adding the flour mixture with the sour cream into the butter-sugar mixture. Beat until combined.

6. Pour the batter into the loaf tin and bake for 50–55 minutes or until a toothpick inserted into the centre comes out clean. Cool completely in the tin. Once cooled, gently turn out of the tin.

7. Drizzle the glaze over the cooled cake. Slice and serve at room temperature with raspberries or strawberries, whipped cream, and a sprinkle of icing sugar (if using).

    Glaze: In a small bowl, whisk all the ingredients together until smooth.

Store it
Store in an airtight container for up to 3 days, or in the freezer – slices separated by sheets of baking parchment – for up to 3 months. Defrost at room temperature.

Tip
Make this into a traditional pound cake by omitting the lemon juice and zest.
You could also then add chocolate chips and make a chocolate chip pound cake.

Makes:
18

Prep time:
25 minutes, plus cooling

Cook time:
35 minutes

If you like pumpkin, you will definitely fall in love with this recipe. The cream cheese frosting adds just the right amount of sweetness to turn the already amazingly moist cupcake into a scrumptious dessert. My youngest son, Rex, can smell these cupcakes being made a mile away, bringing a huge smile to his face.

Rex's Favourite Pumpkin Cupcakes

300g (10oz) golden granulated sugar

140g (5oz) light vegetable oil, such as avocado oil

2 large eggs

225g can 100 per cent pure pumpkin

280g (9½oz) No. 1 All-Purpose Flour Blend (see p24)

½ tsp salt

1 tsp xanthan gum

1 tsp baking powder

½ tsp bicarbonate of soda

½ tsp ground cinnamon

¼ tsp ground allspice

¼ tsp ground nutmeg

⅛ tsp ground cloves

80ml (2¾fl oz) water

For the cream cheese frosting

115g (4oz) salted butter, slightly softened

225g (8oz) cream cheese, chilled and firm

1 tsp vanilla extract

520–650g (1lb 3oz–1lb 7oz) icing sugar, to taste

1–2 tbsp whole milk

1. Preheat the oven to 180°C (160°C fan/350°F/Gas 4) and line the muffin tins with paper cases. In the bowl of a stand mixer fitted with the whisk attachment, or in a large bowl, whisk together the sugar and oil on medium speed until well combined.

2. Add the eggs and whisk on medium-high speed until well combined. Add the pumpkin and whisk on medium speed until well combined.

3. In a separate medium bowl, whisk together the No. 1 All-Purpose Flour Blend, salt, xanthan gum, baking powder, bicarbonate of soda, cinnamon, allspice, nutmeg, and cloves.

4. Alternate adding the dry ingredients and the water into the wet ingredients, starting and ending with the flour mixture. Stir until well combined.

5. Using an ice-cream scoop, fill each muffin case about two-thirds full. Bake for 30–35 minutes or until a toothpick inserted into the centres comes out clean. Cool completely before frosting.

   Cream Cheese Frosting: In a stand mixer fitted with the paddle attachment, or in a large bowl, beat the butter for 1 minute. Add the cream cheese and beat for an additional 2 minutes. Add the vanilla and icing sugar, beat on low speed until combined, and then increase the speed to medium and beat until fluffy, about 5 minutes. Slowly beat in the milk a few teaspoons at a time for about 1 minute, until the desired consistency is reached.

Store it

Store in an airtight container in the refrigerator for up to 5 days. Bring to room temperature before serving.

Tip

To frost the cupcakes, use a piping bag and a large icing tip for the prettiest result. My favourite icing tip is a Wilton 1M open star icing tip.

Makes:
1 x 23cm (9in)
two-tiered cake

Prep time:
30 minutes, plus cooling
and chilling

Cook time:
40 minutes

I've always considered carrot cake to be one of the prettiest cakes, especially when you walk into a café and the layers of cake and cream cheese frosting are staring at you from the case. The secret to this super-moist cake is the pineapple, which also adds the perfect touch of sweetness.

Super-Moist Pineapple Carrot Cake

115g (4oz) salted butter, melted, plus extra for greasing

320g (11oz) No. 1 All-Purpose Flour Blend (see p24), plus extra for dusting

225g can unsweetened crushed pineapple

4 large eggs

120ml (4fl oz) buttermilk

200g (7oz) golden granulated sugar

175g (6oz) light brown sugar

1 tsp vanilla extract

2 tsp apple cider vinegar

2 tsp xanthan gum

2 tsp bicarbonate of soda

2 tsp ground cinnamon

¼ tsp salt

225g (8oz) grated carrots

75g (2¾oz) pecans, chopped, plus extra (optional) for decorating

100g (3½oz) desiccated coconut

1 quantity Cream Cheese Frosting (see left)

1. Preheat the oven to 180°C (160°C fan/350°F/Gas 4). Grease and lightly flour only the bases of 2 x 23cm (9in) round cake tins. Drain the pineapple, reserving 2 tablespoons of its liquid.

2. In a stand mixer fitted with the paddle attachment, or in a large bowl, beat the eggs, buttermilk, butter, granulated sugar, brown sugar, vanilla, and vinegar on medium-high speed until well combined.

3. In a separate medium bowl, whisk together the No. 1 All-Purpose Flour Blend, xanthan gum, bicarbonate of soda, cinnamon, and salt.

4. Gently stir the flour mixture into the wet ingredients. Add the pineapple, 2 tablespoons of the reserved pineapple juice, carrots, pecans, and coconut, and stir until just combined. Let the batter sit for 5 minutes.

5. Stir the batter a couple of times and then pour equal amounts of batter into the 2 prepared cake tins. Bake for 35–40 minutes or until a toothpick inserted into the centres comes out clean. Cool in the tins for 10 minutes, and then invert the cakes out of the tins onto a wire rack and cool completely.

6. Once completely cooled, frost the cake. Place a layer of cake on a serving plate. Spread about 280g (10oz) of frosting on top of the cake, leaving a border of about 1cm (½in) around the edge. Place the second cake on top and press down lightly. Use the remaining frosting to cover the top and sides of the cake. Press chopped pecans into the frosting around the cake for decoration, if desired. Refrigerate until ready to serve.

Store it

Store in an airtight container in the refrigerator for up to 5 days. Bring to room temperature before serving.

Makes:
1 large bundt cake

Prep time:
30 minutes

Cook time:
1¼ hours

Special equipment:
25cm (10in) bundt tin

non-stick cooking spray,
    for greasing
175g (6oz) dark chocolate
280g (9½oz) No. 1
    All-Purpose Flour Blend
    (see p24)
1½ tsp xanthan gum
30g (1oz) cocoa powder
¼ tsp salt
¾ tsp bicarbonate of soda
¾ tsp baking powder
170g (5¾oz) salted butter,
    softened
300g (10oz) golden
    granulated sugar
3 large eggs
1½ tsp vanilla extract
2 tsp apple cider vinegar
3 tbsp chocolate syrup
180ml (6fl oz) buttermilk

For the glaze
120ml (4fl oz) double
    cream
115g (4oz) dark chocolate,
    chopped

This cake is a very impressive and tasty beauty. The richness from using three different chocolates is sure to please the most avid chocolate lover. It's excellent served with strawberries, or vanilla ice cream.

Glazed Triple Chocolate Bundt Cake

1. Place the oven shelf in the lower one-third of the oven and preheat the oven to 160°C (140°C fan/325°F/Gas 3). Generously grease a 25cm (10in) bundt tin with non-stick cooking spray.

2. Melt the dark chocolate and set aside to cool to room temperature.

3. In a medium bowl, whisk together the No. 1 All-Purpose Flour Blend, xanthan gum, cocoa powder, salt, bicarbonate of soda, and baking powder. Set aside.

4. In a stand mixer fitted with the paddle attachment, or in a large bowl, cream the butter and sugar on medium-high speed until light and fluffy, 3–5 minutes.

5. Beat in the eggs one at a time until incorporated. Beat in the vanilla, vinegar, chocolate syrup, and cooled melted chocolate on medium-high speed until incorporated.

6. Reduce the speed to low and alternate adding the dry ingredients and the buttermilk into the wet ingredients, starting and ending with the flour mixture. Mix on medium speed until just combined.

7. Pour the batter into the prepared tin and bake for 60–75 minutes or until the cake springs back when touched and a toothpick inserted into the centre comes out clean. Let cool in pan for 30 minutes and then invert onto a wire rack.

8. While the cake is still slightly warm, drizzle with the glaze, and then cool completely. Slice and serve at room temperature.

Glaze: In a small saucepan, bring the cream just to the boil over a medium heat. Remove from the heat. Add the chopped dark chocolate. Let sit for 5 minutes, and then whisk until smooth.

Store it

Store covered in the refrigerator for up to 3 days, or in individual airtight containers in the freezer for up to 3 months. Defrost at room temperature.

Tip

You can make individual bundt cakes by using mini bundt tins. Depending on the size of your tins, start checking for doneness after 30 minutes.

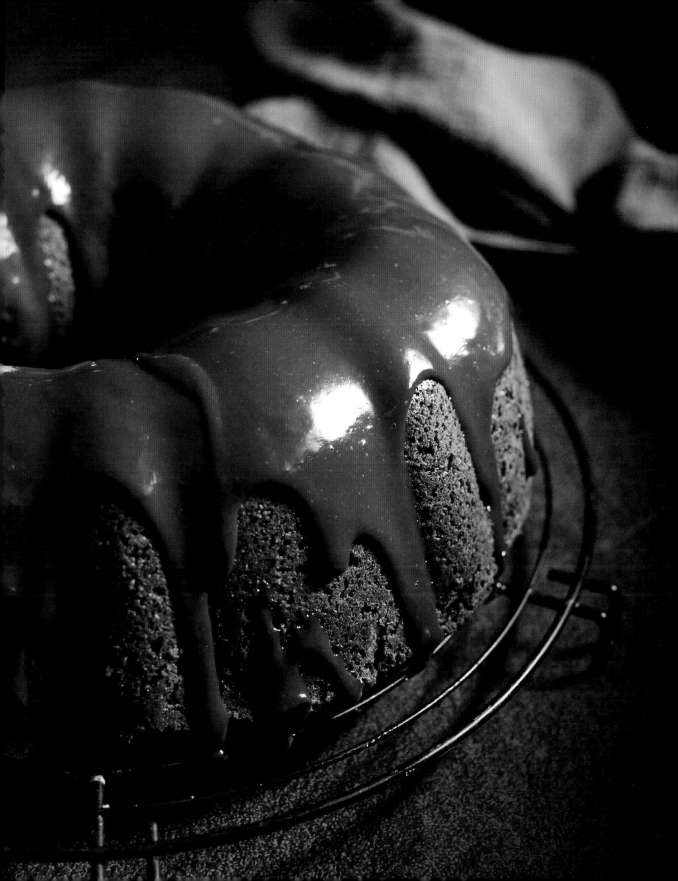

Makes:
1 x 23cm (9in)
two-tiered cake

Prep time:
55 minutes, plus cooling

Cook time:
30 minutes

400g (14oz) No. 1
   All-Purpose Flour Blend
   (see p24)
1 tsp salt
½ tsp bicarbonate of soda
2 tsp baking powder
2 tsp xanthan gum
155g (5½oz) salted butter,
   softened
300g (10oz) golden
   granulated sugar
2 large eggs, at room
   temperature
2 tsp vanilla extract
1 tbsp apple cider vinegar
3 tbsp cocoa powder
1–2 tbsp liquid red food
   colouring or ¾–1 tsp red
   gel food colouring
   (depending on
   desired colour)
2–3 tbsp water
240ml (8fl oz) buttermilk
1 quantity Cream Cheese
   Frosting (see p160)

This red velvet cake not only has a rich flavour, but also a rich, deep colour and layers of cream cheese frosting. It's a beautiful cake for serving on Valentine's Day! It's one of my father-in-law's favourites, so of course I had to create a gluten-free version.

Red Velvet Cake

1. Preheat the oven to 180°C (160°C fan/350°F/Gas 4) and line the bases of 2 x 23cm (9in) round cake tins with baking parchment. Do not grease the sides of the pans.

2. In a medium bowl, sift together the No. 1 All-Purpose Flour Blend, salt, bicarbonate of soda, baking powder, and xanthan gum.

3. In a stand mixer fitted with the paddle attachment, or in a large bowl, beat the butter on medium-high speed for 30 seconds. Beat in the sugar 50g (1¾oz) at a time, scraping down the sides of the bowl as needed after each addition. Once all the sugar has been added, beat for an additional 2 minutes on high speed until light and fluffy. Beat in the eggs one at a time until incorporated. Beat in the vanilla and vinegar.

4. In a bowl, make a paste with the cocoa powder, food colouring, and 2 tablespoons water if using liquid colouring or 3 tablespoons water if using gel colouring.

5. Beat the food colouring paste into the cake batter on low speed. On low speed, alternate beating in the flour mixture and buttermilk, starting and ending with the flour mixture. Mix just until combined; do not overmix. Let sit for 5 minutes.

6. Pour the batter equally into the two prepared cake tins and bake for 25–30 minutes or until a toothpick inserted into the centres comes out clean and the cakes bounce back when touched. Cool in the tins on a wire rack for 10 minutes. Remove the cakes from the tins and cool completely on a rack.

7. Once completely cooled, frost the cake. Place a layer on a serving plate. Spread about 280g (10oz) frosting on top of the cake, leaving a border of about 1cm (½in) around the edge. Place the second cake on top and press down lightly. Use the remaining frosting to cover the top and sides of the cake. Refrigerate until ready to serve.

Store it

Cover with cling film or transfer to an airtight container and store in the refrigerator for up to 3 days.

Tip

You can also use natural food colouring if you prefer, as we do in our house. Our red velvet cake is never the bright red colour you see in shops or restaurants, but it still tastes and looks great. The richness and brightness of colour of your cake will depend on how much food colouring you decide to use.

Makes:
1 x 23cm (9in) two-tiered cake

Prep time:
45 minutes, plus cooling and chilling

Cook time:
50 minutes

For the pastry cream filling

480ml (16fl oz) whole milk

135g (4¾oz) golden granulated sugar

6 large egg yolks

30g (1oz) arrowroot

28g (1oz) salted butter

2 tsp vanilla extract

For the cake

400g (14oz) No. 1 All-Purpose Flour Blend (see p24), plus more for dusting

1 tsp xanthan gum

3 tsp baking powder

½ tsp salt

300ml (10½fl oz) whole milk

150g (5½oz) salted butter

3 large eggs, plus 1 large egg white

300g (10oz) golden granulated sugar

2 tsp apple cider vinegar

2 tsp vanilla extract

For the ganache

115g (4oz) dark chocolate chips

120ml (4fl oz) double cream

I created this recipe for my dad. He's not gluten-free, but Boston Cream Pie is his favourite dessert, and I wanted to create one that the whole family could enjoy. This cake has multiple steps and can be time consuming, but the light buttery cake, creamy vanilla custard, and rich chocolate ganache will be worth every second.

Boston Cream Pie

1. Prepare the pastry cream filling. In a medium saucepan bring the milk and half the sugar to the boil over a medium-high heat. Immediately remove from the heat. In a stand mixer fitted with the paddle attachment, or a large bowl, beat the egg yolks on medium-high speed until light and fluffy, about 1 minute. Add the arrowroot and remaining sugar and beat on medium speed until no lumps remain.

2. Whisk in 60ml (2fl oz) hot milk until combined. Slowly whisk in the remaining milk. Return the mixture to the saucepan over a medium-high heat, whisking, until thickened and gently boiling. Remove from the heat, whisk in the butter and vanilla. Let cool slightly, then cover with cling film. Chill for 4–6 hours.

3. While the filling chills, make the cake. Preheat the oven to 180°C (160°C fan/350°F/Gas 4). Line the bases of 2 x 23cm (9in) round cake tins with baking parchment. Do not grease the sides. In a small bowl, whisk together the No. 1 All-Purpose Flour Blend, xanthan gum, baking powder, and salt. Set aside. In a small saucepan, combine the milk and butter over low heat.

4. While the milk and butter are warming, in a stand mixer fitted with the paddle attachment, or in a large bowl, beat the eggs, egg white, and sugar on high speed until light and fluffy, 4–5 minutes. Whisk in the flour mixture.

5. Increase the heat to medium-high and bring the milk and butter just to the boil, stirring. Add to the batter with the vinegar and vanilla. Whisk until smooth.

6. Pour the batter into the prepared tins and bake for 22–25 minutes or until a toothpick inserted into the centres comes out clean. Cool in the tins on a wire rack for 10 minutes. Remove from the tins and cool completely on a wire rack.

7. Place one cake on a serving plate. Spread the filling on top, leaving a 1cm (½in) border. Place the second cake on top and press down lightly. Refrigerate for 10 minutes. Pour the ganache generously over the cake. Store in the refrigerator to firm up until ready to serve. Serve chilled or at room temperature.

   Chocolate Ganache: Put the chocolate chips in a heatproof bowl. In a small saucepan, bring the cream to the boil over a medium heat, stirring. Pour it over the chocolate and stir until smooth. Drizzle on the cake before it thickens.

Store it ···
Cover and store in the refrigerator for up to 3 days.

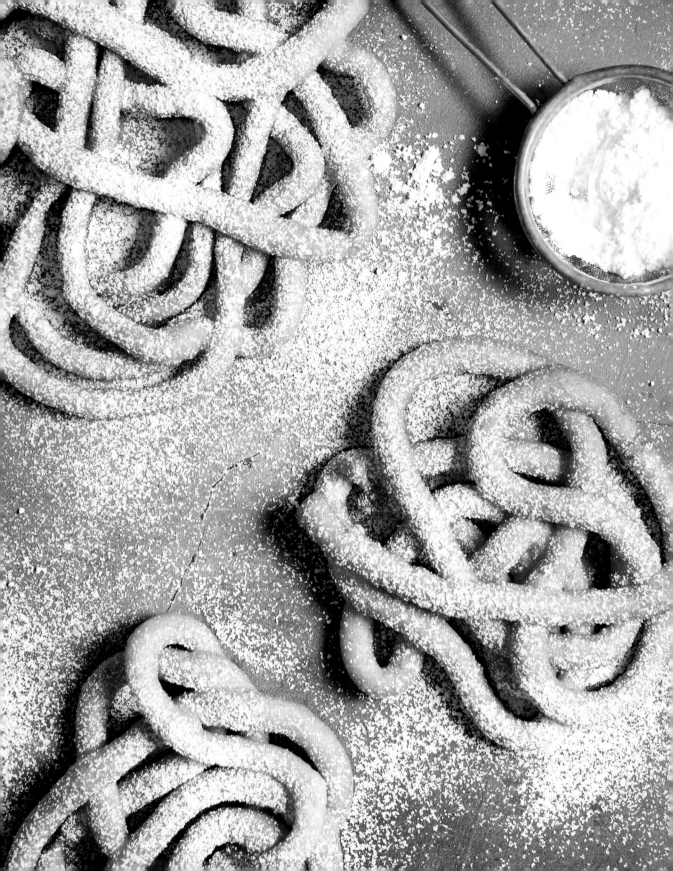

Makes:
15

Prep time:
15 minutes

Cook time:
25 minutes

Special equipment:
cooking thermometer

440–545ml (15–18fl oz)
high smoke-point oil,
such as avocado oil,
for deep-frying

2 large eggs

480ml (16fl oz) whole milk

1 tsp vanilla extract

320g (11oz) No. 1
All-Purpose Flour Blend
(see p24)

1 tsp salt

2 tsp baking powder

2 tsp xanthan gum

2 tbsp golden granulated
sugar

55g (1¾oz) salted butter,
melted

icing sugar, for dusting

This one is for you, Jer! My brother and I LOVE funnel cakes. Occasionally on Saturday mornings when we were growing up, my dad would surprise us with home-made funnel cakes. They were SO good. So, here's my gluten-free version that's light, airy, and delicious.

County Fair Funnel Cakes

1. Line a wire rack with kitchen paper or newspaper. In a large frying pan, preheat 2.5cm (1in) of oil to 180–190°C (350–375°F). (This specific temperature range is important; if the oil is not hot enough, the cakes will absorb too much oil and become dense and soggy.)

2. In a stand mixer fitted with paddle attachment, or in a large bowl, beat the eggs on high speed until light and fluffy, about 1½ minutes. Add the milk and vanilla and beat on low speed until combined.

3. In a separate medium bowl, whisk together the No. 1 All-Purpose Flour Blend, salt, baking powder, xanthan gum, and sugar.

4. On low speed, beat the dry ingredients into the wet ingredients. Increase the speed to medium-high and beat until smooth, scraping down the sides as needed.

5. Fold in the melted butter with a spatula. Fill a squeezy bottle or piping bag with the batter. Creating one funnel cake at a time, squeeze the batter into the hot oil using a circular motion, overlapping the lines of batter to form a net.

6. Fry for 45–60 seconds until light golden brown around the edges, flip, and fry for an additional 45–60 seconds.

7. Carefully remove from the oil and place on the lined wire rack to absorb the oil. Sprinkle liberally with icing sugar and serve immediately. Repeat until you've fried all the batter.

Store it

These are best served immediately and don't reheat or store well.

Tips

This batter is thicker than a traditional gluten-filled batter, which is why you should use a squeezy bottle or piping bag so you can squeeze the batter into the hot oil.

If the batter does not immediately sizzle and float, the oil is not hot enough.

Brownies & Cookies

Makes:
about 60 small squares

Prep time:
30 minutes, plus
2½ hours cooling
and chilling

Cook time:
30 minutes

115g (4oz) salted butter,
melted, plus extra
for greasing

3 large eggs

150g (5½oz) golden
granulated sugar

115g (4oz) light brown
sugar

1 tsp vanilla extract

60g (2oz) cocoa powder

40g (1¼oz) brown rice
flour

50g (1¾oz) ground
almonds

30g (1oz) tapioca flour

1 tsp xanthan gum

¼ tsp salt

For the mint layer

85g (3oz) salted butter,
softened

390g (14oz) icing sugar

1 tsp peppermint extract

6 drops green food
colouring

2 tbsp whole milk, plus
extra if needed

**For the chocolate
ganache**

105g (3½oz) dark
chocolate chips

85g (3oz) salted butter

2 tsp vanilla extract

These remind me of After Eight Mints, or Viscount Mint Creams biscuits, which I desperately miss. They combine chewy brownies with a creamy mint layer and rich chocolate ganache on top. They're outrageously delicious… I bet you can't eat just one.

Mint Brownies

1. Preheat the oven to 180°C (160°C fan/350°F/Gas 4) and lightly grease only the bottom of a 23cm (9in) square tin. In a stand mixer fitted with the paddle attachment, or in a large bowl, beat the eggs on high speed until light and fluffy, about 2 minutes. Add the granulated sugar, brown sugar, melted butter, and vanilla. Beat until well combined.

2. In a separate small bowl, whisk together the cocoa powder, brown rice flour, ground almonds, tapioca flour, xanthan gum, and salt. Slowly stir the dry ingredients into the wet ingredients until well combined.

3. Pour the batter into the prepared tin and bake for 25–30 minutes or until the centre is set. Let cool completely in the tin.

4. Prepare the mint layer. In a stand mixer fitted with the paddle attachment, or in a medium bowl, beat together the butter, icing sugar, peppermint extract, food colouring, and milk on medium-high speed until blended. If it's too thick to spread, add more milk 1 teaspoon at a time until spreadable.

5. Spread the mint layer over the cooled brownies. Cover the tin with cling film and refrigerate for 1 hour.

6. Prepare the chocolate ganache. In a small pan, melt the chocolate chips, butter, and vanilla over a low heat, stirring frequently, until melted and smooth. Remove from the heat and allow the ganache to cool slightly, 1–2 minutes. Gently spread the chocolate ganache over the chilled mint layer.

7. Let the brownies set and chill in the refrigerator for at least 1 hour before cutting. Once chilled, trim the edges, then cut the brownies into 2.5cm (1in) squares and serve chilled or at room temperature.

Store it ··

Store in an airtight container in the refrigerator for up to 1 week, or in the freezer – layers separated by sheets of baking parchment – for up to 3 months. Defrost in the refrigerator or at room temperature.

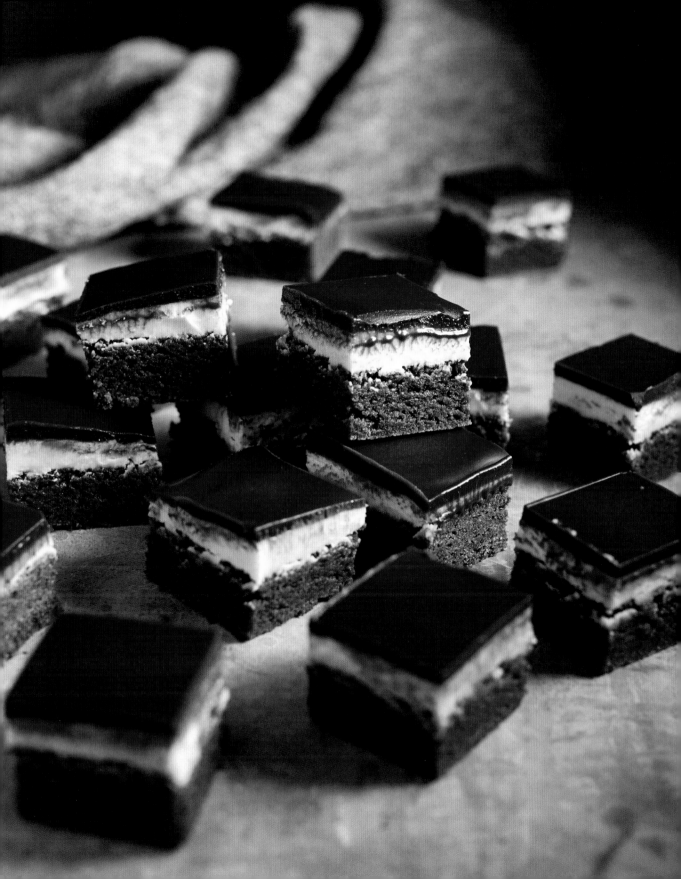

Makes:
9 large squares

Prep time:
15 minutes

Cook time:
30 minutes, plus cooling

3 large eggs

150g (5½oz) golden granulated sugar

115g (4oz) light brown sugar

115g (4oz) salted butter, melted

1 tsp vanilla extract

60g (2oz) cocoa powder

40g (1½oz) brown rice flour

50g (1¾oz) ground almonds

30g (1oz) tapioca flour

1 tsp xanthan gum

¼ tsp salt

Brownies are that universal dessert that just about everyone loves. This version is so rich, chewy, and delicious that no one will believe you when you tell them they are gluten-free. Serve them by themselves, or as part of a brownie sundae with ice cream, chocolate syrup, whipped cream, peanuts, and a cherry on top.

Fudgey Brownies

1. Preheat the oven to 180°C (160°C fan/350°F/Gas 4) and line a 23cm (9in) square tin with baking parchment, leaving some hanging over the sides for easy removal. In a stand mixer fitted with the paddle attachment, or in a large bowl, beat the eggs on high speed until light and fluffy, about 2 minutes.

2. Add the granulated sugar, brown sugar, melted butter, and vanilla. Beat on medium-high speed until well combined.

3. In a separate medium bowl, whisk together the cocoa powder, brown rice flour, ground almonds, tapioca flour, xanthan gum, and salt. Slowly stir the dry ingredients into the wet ingredients until well combined.

4. Pour the batter into the prepared tin and bake for 25–30 minutes or until the centre is set. Let cool completely in the tin. Once cooled, use the overhanging baking parchment to pull the brownies out of the pan. Cut into 7.5cm (3in) squares. Serve at room temperature.

Store it

Store in an airtight container for up to 3 days, or in the freezer for up to 3 months. Defrost at room temperature.

Tip

To make mini brownies, thoroughly grease a mini silicone muffin pan. If you love the corner pieces of brownies, this is the way to go! Once cooled, pop them out and each brownie will have that crispy, chewy edge that the corner pieces have.

Makes:
16 medium-large squares

Prep time:
15 minutes

Cook time:
35 minutes, plus cooling

3 large eggs

150g (5½oz) golden granulated sugar

115g (4oz) light brown sugar

115g (4oz) salted butter, melted

1 tsp vanilla extract

60g (2oz) cocoa powder

40g (1¼oz) brown rice flour

50g (1¾oz) ground almonds

30g (1oz) tapioca flour

1 tsp xanthan gum

¼ tsp salt

150g (5½oz) Reese's Peanut Butter Cups Minis, or regular Reese's Peanut Butter Cups, quartered (see tip, below)

Chocolate and peanut butter have been best friends since the beginning of time, and this recipe combines my rich and chewy chocolate brownie with sweet and salty peanut butter. It's sure to please any chocolate and peanut butter fan.

Peanut Butter Cup Brownies

1. Preheat the oven to 180°C (160°C fan/350°F/Gas 4) and line a 23cm (9in) square tin with baking parchment, leaving some hanging over the sides for easy removal. In a stand mixer fitted with the paddle attachment, or in a large bowl, beat the eggs on high speed until light and fluffy, about 2 minutes.

2. Add the granulated sugar, brown sugar, melted butter, and vanilla. Beat on medium-high speed until well combined.

3. In a separate medium bowl, whisk together the cocoa powder, brown rice flour, ground almonds, tapioca flour, xanthan gum, and salt. Slowly stir the dry ingredients into the wet ingredients until well combined.

4. Gently stir in the peanut butter cups. Pour the batter into the prepared tin and bake for 35 minutes, or until the centre is set. Let cool completely in the tin. Once cooled, use the overhanging baking parchment to pull the brownies out of the tin. Cut into 16 squares. Serve at room temperature.

Store it ··

Store in an airtight container for up to 5 days, or in the freezer – layers separated by sheets of baking parchment – for up to 3 months. Defrost at room temperature.

Tips ··

To avoid the hassle of cutting up Reese's Peanut Butter Cups, I like to use Reese's Peanut Butter Cups Minis and leave them whole. Just be careful with any novelty seasonal shaped Reese's, because they're sometimes not gluten-free. As usual: check the packet.

If you or someone you're baking for cannot have peanut butter, this recipe is also amazing with Pip & Nut Chocolate Almond Butter Cups (available in larger supermarkets, and online).

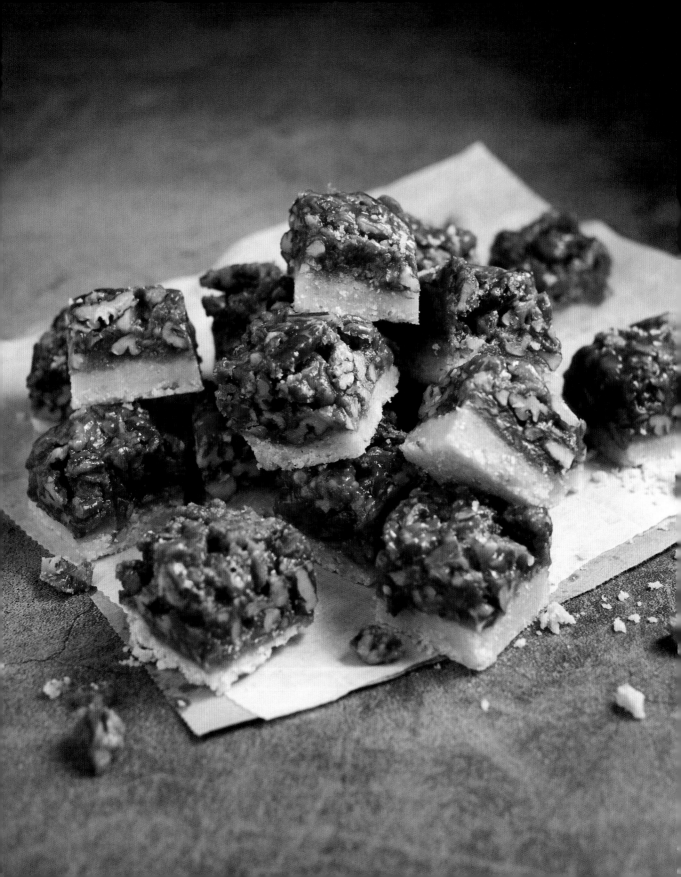

Makes:
about 60 small squares

Prep time:
35 minutes, plus cooling
and chilling

Cook time:
50 minutes

Pecan squares are one of my all-time favourite treats and probably the most-requested of my bakes by family and friends. Even my husband, who rarely eats sweet things, can't resist these, especially when they're placed on top of a bowl of vanilla ice cream.

Irresistible Pecan Squares

For the base

120g (4½oz) No. 1
   All-Purpose Flour Blend
   (see p24)

30g (1oz) arrowroot

60g (2oz) icing sugar

½ tsp salt

1 tsp xanthan gum

115g (4oz) salted butter,
   chilled and cut into
   small pieces

For the filling

170g (6oz) salted butter

85g (3oz) light brown
   sugar

3 tbsp raw honey

½ tsp vanilla extract

pinch of salt

2 tbsp double cream

300g (10oz) pecans,
   chopped

1. Line a 23cm (9in) square baking tin with baking parchment, leaving some hanging over the sides for easy removal. Prepare the base. Put the No. 1 All-Purpose Flour Blend in the bowl of a food processor fitted with the blade attachment, with the arrowroot, icing sugar, salt, and xanthan gum. Pulse a few times to mix.

2. Add the butter. Pulse until pea-sized crumbs are formed. Pour the mixture into the prepared tin and press down very firmly into an even layer. Refrigerate for 15 minutes. Meanwhile, preheat the oven to 180°C (160°C fan/350°F/Gas 4).

3. Remove the base from the refrigerator and bake for 22–25 minutes or until it is set. Let cool while making the filling. (Note, the crust does not need to be completely cooled before adding the filling.)

4. Prepare the filling. Put the butter in a medium saucepan over a medium-low heat with the brown sugar, honey, vanilla, and salt. Stir until the sugar has dissolved and the butter has melted.

5. Increase the heat slightly and bring to the boil. Boil for 3 minutes, constantly stirring and scraping the sides and base of the pan to prevent scorching. Then remove from the heat and stir in the cream and chopped pecans. Immediately pour the pecan mixture over the crust.

6. Bake for 20–25 minutes or until the filling is bubbling and caramel in colour. Place the tin on a wire rack and cool completely. Once cooled, use the overhanging baking parchment to pull the bake out of the pan. Trim the edges, then cut into 2.5cm (1in) squares. Serve at room temperature.

Store it ....

Store in an airtight container in the refrigerator for up to 5 days, or in the freezer – layers separated by sheets of baking parchment – for up to 3 months. Defrost at room temperature or in the refrigerator.

Makes:
16 medium squares

Prep time:
20 minutes, plus cooling

Cook time:
45 minutes

180g (6oz) No. 1 All-Purpose Flour Blend (see p24)

60g (2oz) light brown sugar

60g (2oz) coconut sugar

1 tsp xanthan gum

1 tsp baking powder

¼ tsp salt

125g (4½oz) rolled oats (certified gluten-free)

115g (4oz) salted butter, chilled and cut into pieces

For the fruit filling (optional)

340g jar fruit preserves (any flavour)

For the brown sugar pecan filling (optional)

50g (1¾oz) pecans, chopped

50g (1¾oz) golden granulated sugar

3 tbsp No. 1 All-Purpose Flour Blend (see p24)

1½ tsp ground cinnamon

60g (2oz) salted butter, softened

One huge perk of living in a small community is becoming friends with the people in town. For example, I traded skin treatments for bakes with my beauty therapist, and she asked me to make oat bars. After a few attempts, I created this recipe, which quickly became a hit. Choose between the fruit or brown sugar fillings, or make a batch of both!

Oat Bars

1. To make the brown sugar pecan filling, if using, in a small bowl, combine the pecans, sugar, No. 1 All-Purpose Flour Blend, and cinnamon. Once well combined, using a pastry cutter or your hands, cut in the butter until pea-sized crumbs are formed. Set aside until ready to use.

2. Preheat the oven to 180°C (160°C fan/350°F/Gas 4) and line a 20cm (8in) square baking tin with baking parchment, leaving some hanging over the sides for easy removal. In a large bowl, stir together the No. 1 All-Purpose Flour Blend, brown sugar, coconut sugar, xanthan gum, baking powder, salt, and oats until well combined.

3. Using a pastry cutter or your hands, cut in the butter until evenly distributed. Press half the mixture into the prepared tin.

4. Evenly spread either the fruit filling or the brown sugar pecan filling on top. Sprinkle the remaining oat mixture over the filling and lightly pat down.

5. Bake for 40–45 minutes or until light brown. Let cool completely in the tin. Once cooled, use the overhanging baking parchment to pull the bake out of the tin. Cut into 5cm (2in) squares. Serve at room temperature.

Store it

Store in an airtight container, layers separated by baking parchment, in the refrigerator for up to 3 days, or in the freezer for up to 3 months. Defrost at room temperature.

Makes:
16 medium squares

Prep time:
30 minutes, plus cooling

Cook time:
30 minutes

Chocolate and marshmallow: one of my very favourite flavour combinations. You'll want to make sure you have plenty of napkins nearby, though, because these are a delicious, gooey mess. If you want, add some chopped peanuts on top of these for a little bit of a salty crunch.

S'mores Brownies

3 large eggs
150g (5½oz) golden granulated sugar
115g (4oz) light brown sugar
115g (4oz) salted butter, melted
1 tsp vanilla extract
60g (2oz) cocoa powder
40g (1½oz) brown rice flour
50g (1¾oz) ground almonds
30g (1oz) tapioca flour
1 tsp xanthan gum
¼ tsp salt
150g (5½oz) miniature marshmallows

For the chocolate frosting
115g (4oz) salted butter
80g (2¾oz) cocoa powder
520–585g (1lb 3oz–1lb 5oz) icing sugar
120ml (4fl oz) whole milk

1. Preheat the oven to 180°C (160°C fan/350°F/Gas 4) and line a 23cm (9in) square, deep tin with baking parchment, leaving some hanging over the sides for easy removal. In a stand mixer fitted with the paddle attachment, or in a large bowl, beat the eggs until light and fluffy, about 2 minutes.

2. Add the granulated sugar, brown sugar, melted butter, and vanilla. Beat on medium speed until well combined.

3. In a separate medium bowl, whisk together the cocoa powder, brown rice flour, ground almonds, tapioca flour, xanthan gum, and salt. Slowly stir the dry ingredients into the wet ingredients until well combined.

4. Pour the batter into the prepared tin and bake for 25–30 minutes or until the centre is set. Remove from the oven and immediately spread the marshmallows over the hot brownies. Set aside until cool.

5. Once completely cool, spread the frosting on the brownies. Use the overhanging baking parchment to pull the brownies out of the pan. Cut into 5cm (2in) squares. Serve at room temperature.

Chocolate Frosting: In a medium saucepan, melt the butter. Remove from the heat and stir in the cocoa powder. Stir in 260g (9oz) of the icing sugar. Add the milk and stir until smooth. Stir in enough of the remaining icing sugar to reach a spreadable consistency.

Store it
Store in an airtight container in the refrigerator for up to 5 days, or in the freezer for up to 3 months. Defrost in the refrigerator.

Makes:
about 22

Prep time:
35 minutes, plus
20 minutes chilling

Cook time:
10 minutes

225g (8oz) salted butter, slightly softened

200g (7oz) golden granulated sugar

1 large egg, at room temperature

1 tsp vanilla extract

280g (9½oz) white rice flour

25g (scant 1oz) ground almonds

60g (2oz) tapioca flour, plus extra for dusting

45g (1½oz) potato starch

½ tsp baking powder

2½ tsp xanthan gum

¼ tsp salt

These cookies are soft, buttery, and perfect on their own or decorated with icing. They've become a staple in our home during the holidays, and they work well with cookie cutters of every shape. I like to fill icing bags with different colours of icing and use a very small icing tip to decorate, or simply drizzle on the icing and add some sprinkles.

Sugar Cookies

1. In a stand mixer fitted with the paddle attachment, or in a large bowl, cream the butter and sugar on medium speed until light and fluffy, 3–5 minutes. Add the egg and vanilla and beat well for about 2 minutes.

2. In a separate medium bowl, whisk together the white rice flour, ground almonds, tapioca flour, potato starch, baking powder, xanthan gum, and salt.

3. Slowly add the dry ingredients to the butter mixture and beat on low speed until just combined, scraping down the sides as needed; do not overmix.

4. Form the dough into 2 round discs and wrap in cling film. Refrigerate the dough for at least 10 minutes, or up to 2 days.

5. Preheat the oven to 190°C (170°C fan/375°F/Gas 5) and line a baking tray with baking parchment. Working in batches, on a surface lightly floured with tapioca flour, roll out one of the discs until about 5mm (¼in) thick. Keep the remaining dough in the refrigerator while waiting to be rolled, cut, and baked.

6. Using cookie cutters of your choice, cut the dough into shapes, place on the prepared baking tray, and freeze for 10 minutes.

7. Bake one baking tray at a time for 8–10 minutes. Cool on the baking tray for 5 minutes and then transfer to a wire rack to cool completely. Repeat until all the dough is used and decorate as desired.

Store it

Store undecorated cookies in an airtight container in the freezer. To store decorated cookies, freeze them in a single layer on a baking tray until hardened, then transfer to an airtight container, layers separated by sheets of baking parchment. Freeze for up to 3 months. Defrost in a single layer at room temperature.

Tips

This is a great recipe to make ahead. The longer the cookie dough stays in the refrigerator (up to 2 days), the fluffier the cookies will be.

These cookies are a little fragile when freshly baked. For a sturdier cookie that's easier to decorate, make them one day ahead and store in an airtight container in the freezer.

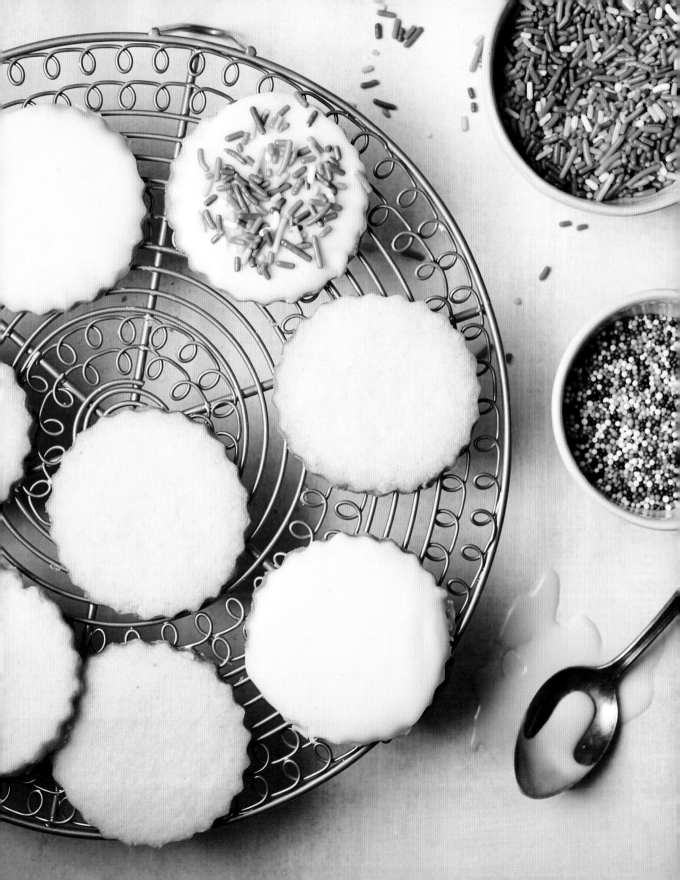

Makes:
about 40

Prep time:
30 minutes, plus chilling and cooling

Cook time:
14 minutes

I have always loved oatmeal cookies because of the texture and all the many different ingredients you can mix in. This recipe includes chewy and plump raisins, but you can always replace them with dried cranberries, or less virtuous chocolate chips, peanut butter cup chips, chopped Daim bar, or any other tiny treat.

Oatmeal Raisin Cookies

115g (4oz) salted butter, softened

100g (3½oz) white vegetable fat (see tip, below)

135g (4¾oz) golden granulated sugar

115g (4oz) light brown sugar

2 large eggs

1 tsp vanilla extract

160g (5¾oz) No. 1 All-Purpose Flour Blend (see p24)

50g (1¾oz) ground almonds

1 tsp bicarbonate of soda

1 tsp ground cinnamon

½ tsp baking powder

2 tsp xanthan gum

½ tsp salt

300g (10oz) rolled oats (certified gluten-free)

150g (5½oz) raisins

1. In a stand mixer fitted with the paddle attachment, or in a large bowl, beat the butter, vegetable fat, granulated sugar, and brown sugar on medium-high speed for 2 minutes.

2. Add the eggs and vanilla and beat on high for 3 minutes more.

3. In a separate medium bowl, whisk together the No. 1 All-Purpose Flour Blend, ground almonds, bicarbonate of soda, cinnamon, baking powder, xanthan gum, salt, and oats.

4. Add the flour mixture to the butter mixture and beat on low speed until just combined. Stir in the raisins. Cover the bowl with cling film and refrigerate for at least 30 minutes.

5. While the dough is chilling, place a shelf in the middle of the oven and preheat the oven to 180°C (160°C fan/350°F/Gas 4). Line a baking tray with baking parchment. Working in batches, scoop heaped tablespoons of cookie dough onto the prepared baking tray about 5cm (2in) apart.

6. Bake in the middle of the oven for 12–14 minutes or until lightly golden brown. Cool on the baking tray for 2–3 minutes and then transfer to a wire rack to cool completely. Repeat with the remaining dough.

Store it

Store in an airtight container for up to 3 days, or in the freezer for up to 3 months. Defrost in the refrigerator or at room temperature.

Tips

Make the dough and refrigerate, tightly covered, up to 24 hours in advance.

Have the cookie dough handy in the freezer to bake just a few at a time. Roll the dough into a log about 5cm (2in) in diameter, wrap well in cling film, and freeze. When ready to bake, unwrap the log and slice off 5mm (¼in) rounds. Place 5cm (2in) apart on the baking tray and bake as instructed.

If you use a brand of vegetable fat that contains a lot of water, you may find your cookies excessively spreading. Chill the dough for at least 1 hour before baking, to help prevent the spreading.

Makes:
about 24

Prep time:
20 minutes, plus cooling

Cook time:
10 minutes

135g (4¾oz) white
    vegetable fat
    (see tip, below)
1 tbsp light vegetable oil,
    such as avocado oil
115g (4oz) coconut sugar
85g (3oz) pure maple
    syrup
75g (2½oz) raw honey
2 tsp vanilla extract
150g (5½oz) ground
    almonds
60g (2oz) arrowroot
28g (1oz) coconut flour
1 tsp salt
1 tsp xanthan gum
½ tsp bicarbonate of soda
2 tsp baking powder
240g (8½oz) dark
    chocolate chips

There was a time when our oldest son was almost 100 per cent refined sugar-, gluten-, and dairy-free. I created this recipe for him. They taste amazing, and you'll want to gobble them all down at once.

Paleo Chocolate Chip Cookies

1. Place a shelf in the middle of the oven and preheat it to 180°C (160°C fan/350°F/Gas 4). Line 2 baking trays with baking parchment. In a stand mixer fitted with the paddle attachment, or in a large bowl, cream together the vegetable fat, oil, coconut sugar, maple syrup, honey, and vanilla on medium-high speed until well combined.

2. Add the ground almonds, arrowroot, coconut flour, salt, xanthan gum, bicarboate of soda, and baking powder. Mix until well combined. Stir in the chocolate chips.

3. Let the dough sit for 10 minutes. Working in batches, scoop heaped tablespoons of cookie dough onto the prepared baking tray about 5cm (2in) apart.

4. Bake one tray at a time in the middle of the oven for 10 minutes, or until golden brown. Let cool on the baking tray for 5 minutes, and then transfer to a wire rack to cool completely. Repeat with the remaining dough.

Store it
Store in an airtight container for up to 3 days, or in the freezer for up to 3 months. Defrost at room temperature, or in the microwave for 30 seconds.

Tip
If you use a brand of vegetable fat that contains a lot of water, you may find your cookies excessively spreading. Chill the dough for at least 1 hour before baking, to help prevent the spreading.

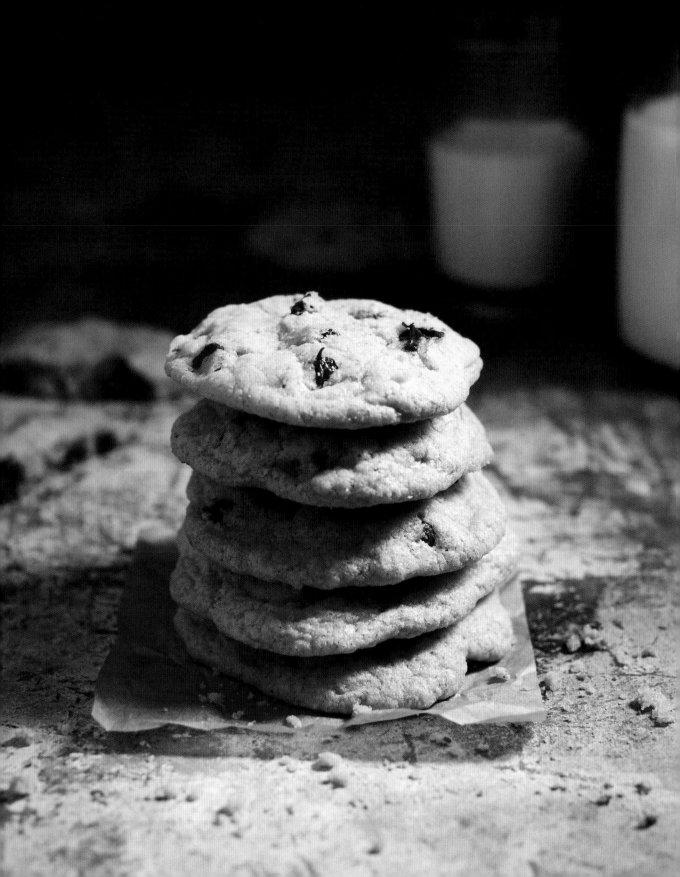

Makes:
about 40

Prep time:
15 minutes, plus chilling
and cooling

Cook time:
15 minutes

115g (4oz) salted butter,
  softened

100g (3½oz) white
  vegetable fat
  (see tip, below)

210g (7½oz) light brown
  sugar

100g (3½oz) golden
  granulated sugar

1 tbsp vanilla extract

2 large eggs, at room
  temperature

320g (11oz) No. 1
  All-Purpose Flour Blend
  (see p24)

50g (1¾oz) ground
  almonds

1 tsp xanthan gum

¾ tsp salt

¾ tsp bicarbonate of soda

400g (14oz) dark
  chocolate chips

I grew up eating freshly baked chocolate chip cookies, and I just had to recreate the recipe. This gluten-free version is about as close as you can get to the original freshly baked cookie of my childhood.

Mum's Famous Chocolate Chip Cookies

1. In a stand mixer fitted with the paddle attachment, or in a large bowl, cream the butter, vegetable fat, brown sugar, and granulated sugar on high speed until light and fluffy.

2. Add the vanilla and eggs and beat on medium-high speed for 3–4 minutes.

3. In a separate medium bowl, whisk together the No. 1 All-Purpose Flour Blend, ground almonds, xanthan gum, salt, and bicarbonate of soda.

4. Slowly add the dry ingredients to the wet ingredients and beat on medium-low speed until combined. Gently stir in the chocolate chips. Refrigerate the dough for at least 1 hour, or up to 2 days.

5. Preheat the oven to 180°C (160°C fan/350°F/Gas 4) and line 2 baking trays with baking parchment. Scoop heaped tablespoons of cookie dough onto the prepared baking tray about 5cm (2in) apart.

6. Bake one tray at a time for 12–15 minutes or until the edges are light brown. Cool completely on a wire rack. Repeat with the remaining dough.

Store it

Store in an airtight container for up to 3 days, or in the freezer for up to 3 months. Defrost at room temperature.

Tips

For a fluffier cookie, refrigerate the dough for at least 1 day. The fat in the dough will solidify when cold, and as the cookies bake, the solidified fat will take longer to melt. The longer the fat remains solid, the less the cookies will spread, so they come out thick and fluffy instead of flat and crunchy.

This dough freezes well. Keep the raw dough balls in an airtight container in the freezer and pop straight into the oven when ready to eat.

If you use a brand of vegetable fat that contains a lot of water, you may find your cookies excessively spreading. Chill the dough for at least 1 hour before baking, to help prevent the spreading.

Makes:
about 45

Prep time:
10 minutes, plus
chilling and cooling

Cook time:
15 minutes

225g (8oz) salted butter,
softened

125g (4½oz) peanut
butter (see tip, below)

340g (12oz) light
brown sugar

2 large eggs

400g (14oz) No. 1
All-Purpose Flour Blend
(see p24)

1 tsp xanthan gum

1½ tsp bicarbonate of
soda

1 tsp baking powder

150g (5½oz) salted
peanuts (optional),
chopped

golden granulated sugar,
for sprinkling

These are slightly crunchy on the outside and chewy on the inside with a perfect mix of sweet and salty. If you cannot have peanut butter, substitute almond butter.

Peanut Butter Cookies

1. Preheat the oven to 180°C (160°C fan/350°F/Gas 4) and line a baking tray with baking parchment. In a stand mixer fitted with the paddle attachment, or in a large bowl, beat the butter, peanut butter, and brown sugar on medium-high speed until creamy. Beat in the eggs one at a time on high speed.

2. In a separate medium bowl, whisk together the No. 1 All-Purpose Flour Blend, xanthan gum, bicarbonate of soda, and baking powder. Stir the dry ingredients into the wet ingredients until just combined. Stir in the peanuts (if using). Refrigerate for at least 30 minutes, or up to 2 days.

3. Working in batches, scoop heaped tablespoons of cookie dough onto the prepared baking tray about 5cm (2in) apart. Keep the remaining dough in the refrigerator until ready to use. Using the tines of a fork, gently press down onto the tops of the balls in a criss-cross pattern. If the fork begins to stick, rinse it off and leave it slightly wet. Sprinkle each cookie with granulated sugar.

4. Bake one tray at a time for 12–15 minutes or until a very light golden brown. Let cool on the baking tray for 3 minutes and then transfer to a wire rack to cool completely. Repeat with the remaining dough.

Store it

Store in an airtight container for up to 3 days, or in the freezer for up to 3 months. Defrost at room temperature, or in the microwave for 25 seconds.

Tip

For peanut-free cookies, replace the peanut butter with almond butter and the peanuts with chopped almonds. For a nut-free version, use sunflower seed butter and sunflower seeds.

Makes:
about 40

Prep time:
30 minutes, plus
chilling and cooling

Cook time:
14 minutes

San Luis Obispo is a Californian city that's home to an incredible cookie shop. When I was in college, I would buy one of their cowboy cookies every week when I went to the farmer's market. It's the best shop-bought cookie I've ever had, so of course I created a gluten-free version. These cookies are chewy, with an incredible mix of flavours.

California Cowboy Cookies

200g (7oz) white
   vegetable fat
   (see tip, below)
100g (3½oz) golden
   granulated sugar
250g (9oz) light brown
   sugar
2 large eggs
1 tsp vanilla extract
200g (7oz) No. 1
   All-Purpose Flour Blend
   (see p24)
100g (3½oz) ground
   almonds
1 tsp bicarbonate of soda
1 tsp xanthan gum
½ tsp salt
½ tsp baking powder
½ tsp ground cinnamon
150g (5½oz) rolled oats
   (certified gluten-free)
150g (5½oz) Daim bar
   pieces
160g (5¾oz) mini
   chocolate chips
50g (1¾oz) desiccated
   coconut

1. Place a shelf in the middle of the oven and preheat it to 180°C (160°C fan/350°F/Gas 4). Line a baking tray with baking parchment. In a stand mixer fitted with the paddle attachment, or in a large bowl, cream the vegetable fat, granulated sugar, and brown sugar on medium-high speed until well combined.

2. Add the eggs and vanilla and beat on medium-high speed for 4 minutes.

3. In a separate medium bowl, whisk together the No. 1 All-Purpose Flour Blend, ground almonds, bicarbonate of soda, xanthan gum, salt, baking powder, and cinnamon. Mix the dry ingredients into the wet ingredients on low speed until just combined.

4. Stir in the oats, Daim bar pieces, chocolate chips, and coconut. Cover the bowl with cling film and refrigerate for at least 1 hour or up to 2 days. (The longer it chills, the fluffier the cookies will be.)

5. Working in batches, scoop heaped tablespoons of cookie dough onto the prepared baking tray about 5cm (2in) apart. Keep the remaining dough in the refrigerator until ready to use.

6. Bake one tray at a time for 12–14 minutes or until just starting to turn golden brown. Cool on the baking tray for 5 minutes and then transfer to a wire rack to cool completely. Repeat with the remaining dough.

Store it ··

Store in an airtight container in the freezer for up to 3 months. Defrost at room temperature, or in the microwave for 20–30 seconds.

Tips ··

You can bake these cookies without refrigerating the dough first. However, chilling the dough for at least 1 hour will yield a slightly fluffier, softer cookie.

If you use a brand of vegetable fat that contains a lot of water, you may find your cookies excessively spreading. Chill the dough for at least 1 hour before baking, to help prevent the spreading.

Makes:
24

Prep time:
30 minutes, plus cooling

Cook time:
17 minutes

My mum made Russian tea cakes every Christmas, and when my first gluten-free Christmas rolled around, I missed them terribly. When local shops asked me to make some special cookies for the holidays, this was the first recipe to pop into my head, and I'm so glad it was. I still look forward to these every year!

Russian Tea Cake Cookies

225g (8oz) salted butter, slightly softened

1 tsp vanilla extract

125g (4½oz) icing sugar, plus 125-250g (4½-9oz) extra for coating

360g (13oz) No. 1 All-Purpose Flour Blend (see p24)

¼ tsp salt

1¼ tsp xanthan gum

150g (5½oz) walnuts or pecans, finely chopped

1. Preheat the oven to 180°C (160°C fan/350°F/Gas 4) and line 2 baking trays with baking parchment. In a stand mixer fitted with the paddle attachment, or in a large bowl, beat the butter and vanilla on high speed for 2 minutes.

2. Add the 125g (4½oz) of icing sugar and beat on medium-high speed for about 5 minutes, scraping down the sides of the bowl halfway through.

3. In a separate small bowl, whisk together the No. 1 All-Purpose Flour Blend, salt, and xanthan gum.

4. Add the flour mixture and the nuts to the butter mixture and beat just until the dough comes together.

5. The dough will be very crumbly and you will need to squeeze it together before rolling. Roll the dough into 4cm (1½in) balls and place on the prepared baking trays about 6cm (2½in) apart. Bake one tray at a time for 15–17 minutes or until just starting to turn brown around the edges.

6. Let cool slightly on the baking trays for 3–4 minutes, but do not cool all the way. Fill a small bowl with the 125–250g (4½–9oz) of icing sugar. While the cookies are still warm, roll them in the icing sugar to coat completely. Set aside to cool completely on a wire rack. Once cooled, roll in the icing sugar for a second coat, and serve.

Store it ··

Store in an airtight container for up to 5 days, or in the freezer for up to 3 months. Defrost at room temperature. You may want to roll the cookies in more icing sugar after they have defrosted.

Tip ···

If your butter gets too soft, or the kitchen is very hot, you can freeze or refrigerate the rolled balls of dough for 5-10 minutes to prevent them from spreading too much.

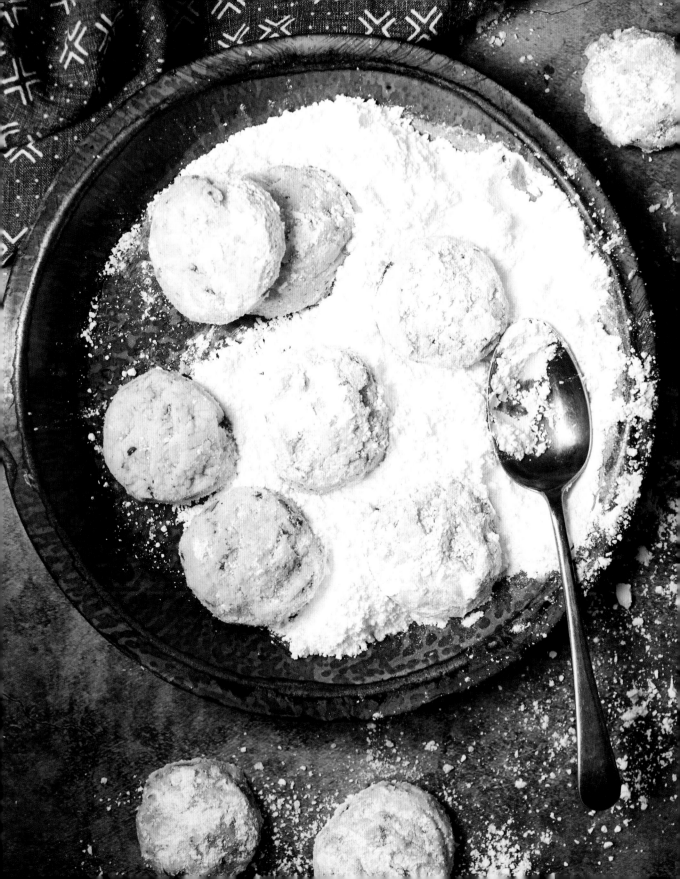

Index

Home-Made Meatballs, 80

horseradish cream sauce, 72

I–J–K

icing sugar doughnuts, 40

Irresistible Pecan Squares, 175

kneading dough, 21

L

labels, reading, 18

leavening agents, 17

Lemon Cupcakes with Raspberry Buttercream, 156

Lemon Pound Cake, 159

Linda's Barbecued Pork Tenderloin, 70

Little Vanilla Scones, 131

Loaded Baked Potato Soup, 99

M

Macadamia Nut Crusted Halibut with Mango Salsa, 44

Mama's Enchilada Pie, 77

mango salsa, 44

Maple Bacon Brussels Sprouts, 88

maple glaze, 40

maple icing, 135

Max's Snickerdoodle Muffins, 125

measuring, 20

Meatloaf with Balsamic Glaze, 83

Meaty Lasagne, 79

Mexican Pizza, 108

Mexican Pork Stew, 101

milk, 19

Mint Brownies, 170

mixing time, 20

Mum's Apple Pie, 139

Mum's Cheesy Potatoes, 92

Mum's Famous Chocolate Chip Cookies, 183

Mum's Famous Meat Sauce, 82

Morning Glory Muffins, 129

muffins
  Blueberry Muffins, 126
  Carrot Courgette Muffins, 128
  crowns, 22
  Grab 'n' Go Cinnamon Streusel Muffins, 130
  Max's Snickerdoodle Muffins, 125
  Morning Glory Muffins, 129

mushiness, 22

N

No. 1 All-Purpose Flour Blend, 24

No. 2 All-Purpose Flour Blend, 24

O

Oat Bars, 176

Oatmeal Raisin Cookies, 180

oils, 19

one-to-one flour blends, 18

Oven "Fried" Chicken, 58

Oven "Fried" Courgettes, 94

P–Q

Paleo Chocolate Chip Cookies, 181

Papa Motte's Pork Fried Rice, 69

Papa's Meaty Chilli, 74

pasta, store-bought, 19

pastry cream filling, 165

Peach Cobbler, 145

Peanut Butter Cookies, 184

Peanut Butter Cup Brownies, 173

Pear Tart, 148

Pecan Pie, 140

personal care products, 18

Phil's Fire Station Beans, 96

pico de gallo, 50

pies
  Buttery Pastry, 138
  Fresh Strawberry Pie, 143
  Mum's Apple Pie, 139
  Pecan Pie, 140
  Pumpkin Pie, 142

pizzas
  Barbecue Chicken Pizza, 105
  Easy Peasy Pizza Crust, 104
  Mexican Pizza, 108
  Thai Chicken Pizza, 107
  Pop's Chicken Wings with Home-Made Ranch Dressing, 52

pork
  BBQ Pork Pizza, 105
  Easy Slow-Cooker Salsa Verde Pork, 67
  Gruyère, Prosciutto, & Chive Scones, 133
  Heavenly Dijon Pork Chops, 66
  Linda's Barbecued Pork Tenderloin, 70
  Maple Bacon Brussels Sprouts, 88
  Mexican Pork Stew, 101
  Papa Motte's Pork Fried Rice, 69
  Pork Chops with Mushroom Gravy, 64

Pork Chops with Mushroom Gravy, 64

potato starch, 16

poultry
  Barbecue Chicken Pizza, 105
  Chicken Parmesan, 54
  Chicken Piccata, 59
  Chicken Salad, 60
  Chicken Shepherd's Pie, 51

Creamy White Chicken Enchiladas, 61

Divine Chicken Divan, 55

Mexican Pizza, 108

Oven "Fried" Chicken, 58

Papa's Meaty Chilli, 74

Pop's Chicken Wings with Home-Made Ranch Dressing, 52

Thai Chicken Pizza, 107

World's Best Chicken Pot Pie, 57

Pumpkin Bread That Started It All, 121

Pumpkin Pie, 142

R

ranch dressing, 52

raspberry buttercream frosting, 156

reading labels, 18

reading recipes, 22

Red Velvet Cake, 164

resting, batters and doughs, 21

Rex's Favourite Pumpkin Cupcakes, 160

Roasted Tenderstem Broccoli, 86

roasted garlic, 91

Russian Tea Cake Cookies, 186

S

scones
  Afternoon Tea Blueberry Scones, 134
  Coffee Shop Maple Scones, 135
  Flaky Sour Cream Scones, 38
  Gruyère, Prosciutto, & Chive Scones, 133
  Little Vanilla Scones, 131

seafood and fish
  Baja Fish Tacos, 50
  Cracklin' Crab Cakes, 47

About the Author

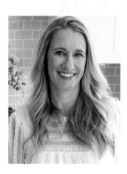

Jennifer Fisher is a gluten-free recipe developer. When she went gluten-free in 2009, she was determined to make all those foods she still loved. So, she dedicated her time to experimenting endlessly in the kitchen, which turned into a small baking business selling gluten-free bakes to a few local shops. Labels aside, customers would never guess her scrumptious treats were gluten-free! The business quickly became a raving success, and she received orders from local health food markets and coffee shops, as well as requests to bake for private parties and gatherings. She ultimately closed her business to focus on her family, but her community never stopped asking about her delicious treats. Jennifer wrote them all down in her first cookbook, *Surprise! It's Gluten-Free!* She lives in San Clemente, a small beach town in Southern California, with her husband Kirk, their two sons Max and Rex, and their dog Fletch.

Author Acknowledgments

This book has been a group effort and would never have been published without the encouragement, love, and support of so many people. Writing a book and caring for two boys is not an easy task, but my in-laws and parents helped me to get it all done. Thank you CP, Linda, Mum, and Dad for your countless hours of driving our boys to wherever they needed to go when I would call in a panic because I had loaves of bread in the oven, for washing mountains of dishes, for baking with me in the kitchen, and – most of all – for eating all my creations!

When I set out to write my first cookbook, I was extremely overwhelmed. I knew how to develop recipes and write them down, but I had no idea how to transform them into a manuscript worthy of sending to a publisher. Mikal Belicove, you worked miracles and turned my recipes written down on scraps of paper into an actual manuscript! Thank you for believing in me, for taking on this project, and for convincing others that I'm worth investing in. This book would definitely not be in existence without you. Thank you, friend!

Alexandra Andrzejewski, my editor, has been a complete joy to work with! Thank you for guiding me, encouraging me, teaching me, and most of all for your kindness and patience. This book would never be what it is without you! Thank you also to the creative team who brought my recipes to life, including Rebecca Batchelor, Lovoni Walker, Ashley Brooks, and Kelley Schulyer.

My mum is a special lady to whom I owe an endless amount of thanks. Not only did she teach me how to cook from a very young age, but she was also the inspiration and original author of so many recipes in this book. Thank you for the hours and hours you spent in the kitchen with me cooking and baking so I could meet my deadlines. You are always there when I need you. Dad, thank you for the many hours you spent entertaining the boys so I could cook and meet deadlines. And thank you for being willing to test every recipe I ever created!

Everything I do, I do for my boys. Thank you Max and Rex for being the most patient and loving two boys for whom a mum could ever ask. You are my biggest inspirations and I love you both more than you could ever imagine. Max, you have believed in me from day one and have always been my number one fan. You are the best taste tester I could ever have. I will never stop creating recipes for you!

This book would not be in existence without my husband. He always believed in me even when I didn't believe in myself. My number one job is to be a wife and mother, but with his encouragement and endless hours of washing dishes and staying up late to take the last batch of cookies out of the oven, I have been able to pursue my passion for helping others with restricted diets. Thank you for being my everything and for all of the selfless acts you do for the boys and me. You are my number one, and I love you.